MEDITATION IS NOT WHAT YOU THINK

ALSO BY JON KABAT-ZINN

FALLING AWAKE: How to Practice Mindfulness in Everyday Life
THE HEALING POWER OF MINDFULNESS: A New Way of Being
MINDFULNESS FOR ALL: The Wisdom to Transform the World

MINDFULNESS:
Diverse Perspectives on Its Meaning, Origins, and Applications
(editor, with J. Mark G. Williams)

MINDFULNESS FOR BEGINNERS:
Reclaiming the Present Moment—and Your Life

THE MIND'S OWN PHYSICIAN:
A Scientific Dialogue with the Dalai Lama on the Healing Power of
Meditation
(editor, with Richard J. Davidson)

LETTING EVERYTHING BECOME YOUR TEACHER:
100 Lessons in Mindfulness

ARRIVING AT YOUR OWN DOOR:
108 Lessons in Mindfulness

THE MINDFUL WAY THROUGH DEPRESSION:
Freeing Yourself from Chronic Unhappiness
(with Mark Williams, John Teasdale, and Zindel Segal)

COMING TO OUR SENSES:
Healing Ourselves and the World Through Mindfulness

EVERYDAY BLESSINGS:
The Inner Work of Mindful Parenting
(with Myla Kabat-Zinn)

WHEREVER YOU GO, THERE YOU ARE:
Mindfulness Meditation in Everyday Life

FULL CATASTROPHE LIVING:
Using the Wisdom of Your Body and Mind to Face Stress, Pain, and Illness

MEDITATION IS NOT WHAT YOU THINK

Mindfulness and Why It Is So Important

JON KABAT-ZINN

hachette
BOOKS

NEW YORK   BOSTON

Hachette Books
Hachette Book Group
1290 Avenue of the Americas
New York, NY 10104
hachettebooks.com
twitter.com/hachettebooks

Originally published in hardcover as part of *Coming to Our Senses* by Hyperion in January 2005.

First Edition: May 2018

Credits and permissions appear beginning on p. 179 and constitute a continuation of the copyright page.

Hachette Books is a division of Hachette Book Group, Inc.
The Hachette Books name and logo are trademarks of Hachette Book Group, Inc.

The publisher is not responsible for websites (or their content) that are not owned by the publisher.

The Hachette Speakers Bureau provides a wide range of authors for speaking events. To find out more, go to www.hachettespeakersbureau.com or call (866) 376-6591.

Library of Congress Control Number: 2018931144

ISBNs: 978-0-316-41174-5 (trade paperback), 978-0-316-52202-1 (ebook)

Printed in the United States of America

LSC-C

10 9 8 7 6 5 4 3 2

for Myla
for Stella, Asa, and Toby
for Will and Teresa
for Naushon
for Serena
for the memory of Sally and Elvin
and Howie and Roz

and for all those who care

for what is possible

for what is so

for wisdom

for clarity

for kindness

for love

CONTENTS

What Is Meditation Anyway?

It is not uncommon for people to think they know what meditation is, especially since it is so much in the common parlance now and images and passing references to it, as well as podcasts and online summits on the subject, abound. But actually and quite understandably, most of us still may be harboring fairly narrow or incomplete perspectives on what meditation is and what it can do for us. It is all too easy to fall into certain stereotypes, such as that meditation is limited to sitting on the floor while effectively banishing all thoughts from one's mind; or that it must be practiced for long periods of time and often, for it to have any positive effect; or that it is inextricably linked to adopting a specific belief system or spiritual framework from an ancient tradition. People may also think that it has almost magical benefits for our bodies, our minds, and our souls. None of this is really the case, although there are elements of truth in all of it. The reality is much more interesting.

So what is meditation, really? And why might it make a lot of sense to at least experiment with bringing it into your life? This is exactly the subject of this book.

Meditation Is Not What You Think was originally published in 2005 as part of a larger book entitled *Coming to Our Senses: Healing Ourselves and the World Through Mindfulness*. Since its initial publication, mindfulness has improbably gone mainstream in a big way. Millions of people around the world have taken up a formal mindfulness meditation practice as part of their everyday lives. To my mind this is a very positive and promising development, one that I had hoped for and have tried to help catalyze over the years along with many other people, in spite of the fact that along with this entering into the mainstream, there inevitably comes some degree of hype, commercial exploitation, opportunism, and people claiming to teach it who have little or no background or training in it. Still, even the hype can be seen as a sign of success, although hopefully one that will be relatively short-lived and contained, as the significant healing and transformative power of mindfulness as a practice and as a way of being in relationship with our lived experience becomes more widely understood and adopted.

While meditation is not all about sitting still on the floor or in a chair, taking your seat both literally and metaphorically is an important element of mindfulness. We could say that in essence, it is a direct and very convenient way to cultivate greater intimacy with your own life unfolding and with your innate capacity to be aware—and to realize how valuable, overlooked, and underappreciated an asset that awareness actually is.

A Love Affair with Life

The act of taking your seat in your own life, which could also be seen as taking a stand of a certain kind, on a regular basis, is in and of itself a profound expression of human intelligence. Ultimately it is a radical act of sanity and love—namely to stop all the doing that carries us *through* our moments without truly inhabiting them, and actually drop into being, even for one fleeting moment. That dropping in is the exceedingly simple, but at the same time, hugely radical act undergirding mindfulness as a meditation practice and as a way of being. It is easy to learn. It is easy to do. But it is also equally easy to forget to practice, even though this kind of dropping in takes literally no time at all, just remembering.

Happily, this intimacy with our own capacity for awareness is increasingly being taken up and nurtured in one form or another by more and more people as it makes its way into various domains of society: from school children to elders, from academics to business professionals, from tech engineers to community leaders and social activists, from college students to medical and graduate students, from—believe it or not—politicians, to athletes at all levels of sport. And for the most part, mindfulness is being nurtured and cultivated not as a luxury or passing fad but with the growing recognition that it may be an absolute necessity for living life fully and for living life with integrity—in other words, ethically—in the face of the starkly looming challenges we are all confronted with every day and with the equally enormous and compelling opportunities and options that are available to us as well at this particular moment in time—that is, if we can see through and transcend at least for a moment, our mind's own self-constructed and habitual limitations, the narratives we tell ourselves that are not true enough if they are true at all, and our endemic blindnesses. This enterprise is ultimately one big and extremely vital adventure—full of ups and downs, just as life itself is full of ups and downs. But how we choose to be in relationship to it makes all the difference in how this adventure, the adventure of your life, unfolds. And you have a lot more say in it than you might suspect.

There are many different ways to cultivate mindfulness through both formal meditation practice and in everyday living and working. As you will see, formal meditation can be practiced in any number of positions: sitting, lying down, standing, or walking. And what we call *informal meditation practice*, which when all is said and done is the real meditation practice, involves letting life itself become coextensive with your meditation practice and recognizing that everything that unfolds within it, the wanted and the unwanted and the unnoticed, is the real curriculum. When we see meditation in this big way, nothing that arises in our own mind or in our own life or in the world is excluded, and any moment is a perfect moment to bring awareness to what is unfolding and thereby learn and grow and heal.

Over time, what is most important is for you to find your own authentic way to practice, a way that feels intuitive and trustworthy, that is true for you while at the same time staying true to the essence of the ancient traditions out of which mindfulness emerged. This book is aimed to help you to do just that, or at least to get started on this lifelong adventure. You will learn how to develop a daily mindfulness practice if it is new to you, or hopefully, to deepen your practice if you already have one. In either case, you will also learn how to see it as a love affair rather than as a chore or a burden, one more "should" in your already-too-busy day, and so, ultimately, a deep inhabiting of the life that is yours to live. As decades of research have shown, mindfulness can serve as a powerful ally in facing and transcending the challenges of stress, pain, and illness throughout life.

Doing and Non-doing

Sometimes being mindful looks like doing something. And sometimes being mindful looks like doing nothing. From the outside, you can't always know. But even when it looks or feels like doing nothing, it isn't. In fact, it isn't a *doing* at all. I know this sounds a bit crazy but mindfulness meditation is much more a matter of non-doing, of simply dropping into *being* in the only moment we ever have—this one—than it is of doing something or getting someplace. How you are—and wherever you are in any moment—is good enough, at least for now! In fact, it is perfect, if you are willing to hold the moment in awareness while being gentle with yourself and not forcing things.

The regular practice of mindfulness meditation helps us to access within ourselves the openhearted spaciousness characteristic of pure awareness and to express it in how we act in the world. Mindfulness as a regular practice can literally and figuratively give your life back to you, especially if you are stressed or in pain, or caught up in uncertainty and emotional turmoil—which of course, we all are to one degree or another in some moments or times in our lives.

But, in spite of its trendy popularity or notoriety at this moment, mindfulness is above all *a practice*, and at times, an arduous one. For most of us, it requires intentional and ongoing cultivation. And that cultivation is nurtured through the regular disciplined practice of meditation, pure and simple. And simple it is, although not necessarily easy at times. That is one of the reasons that it is worth doing. The investment of time and energy is profoundly beneficial. It is healing. It can be totally transformative. That is one of the reasons people often say that the practice of mindfulness "gave me back my life."

Mindfulness Goes Mainstream

There are a lot of different reasons why meditation practice, and in particular, mindfulness meditation, has moved into the mainstream over the past forty plus years. One has to do with the work of an ever-growing community of colleagues from around the world that I have been privileged to be a part of who teach MBSR (mindfulness-based stress reduction), a program that I developed and launched in 1979 at the University of Massachusetts Medical Center. Over the ensuing years, MBSR has inspired the development and study of other mindfulness-based practices such as MBCT (mindfulness-based cognitive therapy) for depression, and a range of other programs modeled on MBSR for other circumstances that people find themselves in, and which have been shown through scientific research to be valuable and effective.*

The original aim of the MBSR clinic, an eight-week outpatient program in the form of a course, was to test the potential value of training in mindfulness to help reduce and relieve the suffering associated with the stress, pain, and illnesses of medical patients with chronic conditions who were not responding to the usual medical

---

* A partial list includes MBCP (mindfulness-based childbirth and parenting); MBRP (mindfulness-based relapse prevention) for binge drinking; MB-EAT (mindfulness-based eating awareness therapy) for disordered eating; MBSPE (mindfulness-based sport performance enhancement); MBWE (mindfulness-based wellness education); etc.

treatments and therefore falling through the cracks of the mainstream medical and health care system. MBSR was meant to be a safety net to catch them as they were falling and challenge them to do something for themselves to participate in their own trajectory toward greater health and well-being, starting from where they found themselves. MBSR was not meant to be a new medical treatment or therapy. Rather, it was meant to be a self-educational public health intervention that over time, as more and more people went through it in large numbers, might have the potential to move the bell curve of humanity in the direction of greater health, well-being, and wisdom. We were in some sense teaching people how to collaborate with whatever their physicians and the hospital could do for them by mobilizing their own interior resources through mindfulness practice and seeing if by doing so, they could stay out of the hospital, or at least use it much more sparingly as they learned to take better care of themselves and develop new ways of effectively dealing with and modulating their levels of stress and pain and their various health challenges and chronic conditions.

We were interested in seeing and documenting as best we could whether meditative practices emphasizing mindfulness, practiced regularly for 45 minutes a day, six days a week over the eight weeks of the program would make a significant difference in the quality of life and in the health and well-being of the participants. For the majority, there was no question right from the start that it did. We could actually see the changes in people over the eight weeks ourselves. They happily shared in class some of the changes they were experiencing and felt empowered by, and our data collection confirmed this.

We began sharing our findings in papers in the medical literature, starting in 1982. Within a few years, other scientists and clinicians took up the increasingly rigorous study of mindfulness as well, adding to the now extensive body of knowledge on this subject in the scientific community.

Today, there is a flourishing exploration of mindfulness and its potential uses in medicine, psychology, neuroscience, and many other fields. In and of itself, this is quite remarkable because it represents the confluence of two domains of human knowledge that have never before encountered each other: medicine and science on the one hand, and ancient contemplative practices on the other.

When *Coming to Our Senses* was published in January of 2005, there were only 143 papers published at that time in the medical and scientific literature that had the word "mindfulness" in the title. That represents 3.8 percent of the 3,737 papers published on mindfulness through 2017. In the interim, an entire field has emerged in medicine and in science more broadly, looking at its effects on everything from our brain's remarkable capacity to reshape itself (what is called *neuroplasticity*), to its effects on our genes and their regulation (what is called *epigenetics*), on our telomeres and thus, on biological aging, and on our thoughts and emotions (especially in terms of depression, anxiety, and addiction), as well as on family life, work life, and our social lives.

A New Format for a New Time

I mentioned earlier that *Meditation Is Not What You Think* was originally published in 2005 as part of a larger book, *Coming to Our Senses*. Given everything that has transpired since, I thought that it might be useful to divide that book into four shorter volumes for a new generation of readers. Since you are holding the first of those books in your hands right now, I am guessing that you must be at least a bit curious about meditation in general and mindfulness in particular to have picked it up and read this far. But even if you are not that curious, or it scares you a bit to think about adding meditation to your life—one more thing that you are going to have to do or that would take up time, precious moments you don't think you have, or you are concerned about what your family and friends might think, or even if the very idea of formal meditation turns you off or seems farfetched and impractical—no need to worry. That is not a problem. Because meditation, and in particular mindfulness meditation, truly is not what you think.

But what meditation can do is transform your relationship to your thinking. It can help you befriend that capacity as one, but only one, of a number of different intelligences you already have and can put to use rather than be imprisoned by, as we so often are by our thoughts when we forget that they are merely thoughts, events in the field of awareness, rather than the truth. So you might say that this book covers the *what* and the *why* of mindfulness.

The next book in the series, *Falling Awake*, explores in detail how to go about systematically cultivating mindfulness in your everyday life. The healing and transformative power of mindfulness lies in the practice itself. Mindfulness is not a technique. It is a way of being in wise relationship to the entirety of your inner and outer experience. And that means that your senses, all of them—and there are far more than five, as you will see—play a huge and critical role. So we could say that this second book covers the *how* of mindfulness in detail, both as a formal meditation practice and as a way of being.

The third book, *The Healing Power of Mindfulness*, is really about the *promise* of mindfulness. It explores the potential benefits of mindfulness from a very broad perspective, including two studies that I was directly involved with. I have not fully documented the results of all the new scientific studies that have come out since 2005. That would be overwhelming, and more are coming out every day. But the major trends are summarized in the foreword to that volume, with references to books describing some of the most exciting recent research.

Beyond the science, this third book in the series also evokes some of the beauty and the poetry inherent in a whole range of perspectives and circumstances that might be both illuminating and healing for us. Some are based on meditative traditions, in particular Zen, Vipassana, Dzogchen, and Hatha Yoga that personally touched me deeply and propelled me to integrate mindfulness into my own life beginning when I was twenty-one years old. They all point to the value of embodied wakefulness and of our intrinsic interconnectedness. Their powerful perspectives, insights, and practices have been transmitted down to us over the centuries—a remarkable human lineage that is very much alive and flourishing today.

The fourth book, *Mindfulness for All*, is about the *realization* of mindfulness in your own life—realization in the sense of making it real and embodying it as best you can in your own way, not just as an individual but as a member of the human family. This book focuses less on the body and more on the body politic and what we have learned in medicine over the past forty years and in the contemplative traditions over the past several thousand years that might be of essential value to us as *Homo sapiens sapiens* at this moment on the planet. It also evokes your own potential as a unique living and breathing human being and your place in the larger world when you persist in inhabiting your own capacity for wakefulness and taste the creativity, generosity, caring, ease, and wisdom doing so naturally gives rise to. So this volume includes not only individual realization, but also a more societal and species-wide waking up to our full potential as human beings.

My hope with these four books is to introduce a new generation to the timeless power of mindfulness and the many different ways in which it can be described, cultivated, and applied in the world as we find it today. In fact, I trust that many new applications and approaches will be developed and implemented by future generations in their own ways, appropriate to the circumstances they will find themselves in. Today, those circumstances include a new awareness of global warming, the unconscionable human costs and the destructiveness of war, institutionalized economic injustice, racism, sexism, agism, implicit bias, sexual harassment and assault, bullying, the challenges of gender identity, cyber-hacking, endless competition for our attention—the so-called "attention economy"—an overall lack of civility, and extreme polarization and demagoguery in government and between governments, along with all of the other horrors as well as the exquisite beauty that have always been part of life unfolding with us humans since the dawn of history.

At the same time, and it is important to keep this perspective in mind as well, nothing has really changed. As the French are fond of saying, *"Plus ça change, plus s'est la meme chose."* The more things change, the more they stay the same. Greed, hatred, and delusion have been operating since the dawn of time in the human mind, and have given rise to endless violence and suffering. So we have our work cut out for us in this moment on the planet, that is, if you choose this path for your own sake and for the sake of the world. At the same time, when the human mind knows itself in a deep way, we have also known beauty, kindness, creativity, and insight since the dawn of time. Generosity and kindness, tenderness and compassion have also always been an essential part of human nature and the human condition, as have transcendent works of art, music, poetry, science, and the possibility of wisdom and of inner and outer peace prevailing.

The Power of the Present Moment When Embraced in Awareness

There is no question that mindfulness, compassion, and wisdom are more important than ever before—even though the essence of mindfulness is and has always been timeless, having to do with our *relationship* to this moment and to any moment as it is, however it is. The past is only available to us in this present moment. And so is what is yet to unfold in a future we try endlessly to envision and control. If you want the future to be different, the only leverage you have is to inhabit the present moment fully, and that means mindfully and heartfully. That itself is an action, even though it looks like non-doing. Then, the very next moment will be full of new possibilities because you were willing to show up in this one. Inhabit this moment fully and the very next moment (the future) is already different. Each moment of now is a branch point. Anything can unfold in the next moment. But what unfolds depends on whether and to what degree you are willing to show up fully awake and aware in this one. Of course it is important at times to take action in the service of wisdom and compassion and justice and freedom. But actions themselves can be mindless or ineffective unless we let our doing come out of our being. Then an entirely different form of doing emerges...what we could call "wise doing," or "wise action," an authentic doing molded in the furnace of mindfulness.

If you check your watch, you will always find, wonder of wonders, that it is now again. What better time to take up mindfulness as a practice and as a way of being, and by doing so, begin or resume or re-energize a lifelong journey of learning, growing, healing, and transformation? At the same time, paradoxically, you will be going nowhere, since you are already whole, already complete, already who you are in your fullness. Mindfulness is not and cannot be about *improving* yourself, because you are already whole, already complete, already perfect (including all your "imperfections"). Rather, it involves *recognizing* that you are already whole, already complete in this very moment, in spite of any counter-arguments that some clever part of your thinking mind might be mobilizing in this very same moment. It is about reclaiming the full dimensionality and possibility of the one life that is yours to live while you have the chance. And then embodying it in one or more of a potentially infinite number of creative ways that will inevitably collapse down in any and every moment into how it actually unfolds in that moment in awareness. There is tremendous freedom of choice and creativity in this way of being both awake and aware moment by moment by moment in our lives.

An Evolutionary Arc

The practice of mindfulness dates back thousands of years in the civilizations of India and China, even predating the Buddha, although it was the Buddha and those who followed in his footsteps over the centuries who articulated it most clearly and in the greatest detail. The Buddha spoke of mindfulness as "the direct path" to liberation from suffering. As we have seen, mindfulness can be thought of as a way of being, one that is continually reexamining and rearticulating the essence of human wakefulness and how it might be embodied in new times and cultures and in the face of new challenges. The word "mindfulness" is coming to represent an evolutionary arc of human wisdom that has been developing for centuries and is now finding new ways and taking on new forms to help us recognize the intrinsic wholeness of our lives as highly interconnected planetary beings, and thus, nurturing the ongoing development of our exceedingly young and highly precocious species. Through ongoing research and exchanges and dialogue between scientists and contemplatives, and through the work of an increasingly large number of diverse, dedicated, and well-trained mindfulness teachers from many different traditions and cultures, we humans are finding ever-more-valid ways to understand mindfulness and its potentially healing and transformative effects, as well as new ways to implement them in different domains. Even politicians and governments around the world are beginning to take notice and engage in its cultivation and practice and develop policies based on its potential to galvanize the health of a community or a nation—not that we should put too much stock in politicians, except that they are human beings too, and are capable of acting for the greater good under some circumstances in ways that could be hugely helpful to those who are systematically disenfranchised and disempowered in society.

The Challenge and the Aspiration

In the end, you might say that the most important challenge is for all of us to wake up at least a little bit more, and to come to our senses both literally and metaphorically to whatever degree we can and to whatever degree we care to, especially if we do realize that mindfulness is fundamentally a love affair with what is deepest and best in ourselves as human beings. Then we will be in a better position to see what is here to be seen, to feel what is here to be felt, to become more aware via all our senses. All of human experience is waiting to be invited more fully into your life, to be held in awareness and, as the experiment or adventure of a lifetime, to see what might unfold while you have the chance. Welcome to an increasingly expanding circle of intentionality and embodied wakefulness.

May your interest in and understanding of mindfulness grow and flower, nourishing and enlivening your life and work, your family and community, and this world we all belong to, from moment to moment and from day to day.

Jon Kabat-Zinn
Northampton, MA
January 24, 2018

INTRODUCTION
THE CHALLENGE OF A LIFE'S TIME—
AND A LIFETIME

It may be when we no longer know what to do,
we have come to our real work,
and that when we no longer know which way to go,
we have begun our real journey.

WENDELL BERRY

I don't know about you, but for myself, it feels like we are at a
critical juncture of life on this planet. It could go any number of different ways. It seems that the world is on fire and so are our hearts,
inflamed with fear and uncertainty, lacking all conviction, and often
filled with passionate but unwise intensity. How we manage to see
ourselves and the world at this juncture will make a huge difference
in the way things unfold. What emerges for us as individuals and as a
society in future moments will be shaped in large measure by whether
and how we make use of our innate and incomparable capacity for
awareness in this moment. It will be shaped by what we choose to do
to heal the underlying distress, dissatisfaction, and outright dis-ease
of our lives and of our times, even as we nourish and protect all that is
good and beautiful and healthy in ourselves and in the world.

The challenge as I see it is one of coming to our senses, both individually and as a species. I think it is fair to say that there is considerable movement in that direction worldwide, with little noticed

and even less understood rivulets and streams of human creativity and goodness and caring feeding into growing rivers of openhearted wakefulness and compassion and wisdom, even in the face of the many challenges the world is facing. Where the adventure is taking us as a species, and in our individual private lives, even from one day to the next, is unknown. The destination of this collective journey we are caught up in is neither fixed nor predetermined, which is to say there is no destination, only the journey itself. What we are facing now and how we hold and understand this moment shapes what might emerge in the next moment, and the next, and shapes it in ways that are undetermined and, when all is said and done, undeterminable, mysterious.

But one thing is certain: This is a journey that we are all on, everybody on the planet, whether we like it or not; whether we know it or not; whether it is unfolding according to plan or not. Life is what it is about, and the challenge of living it as if it really mattered. Being human, we always have a choice in this regard. We can either be passively carried along by forces and habits that remain stubbornly unexamined and which imprison us in distorting dreams and potential nightmares, or we can engage in our lives by waking up to them and participating fully in their unfolding, whether we "like" what is happening in any moment or not. Only when we wake up do our lives become real and have even a chance of being liberated from our individual and collective delusions, diseases, and suffering.

Years ago, a meditation teacher opened an interview with me on a ten-day, almost entirely silent retreat by asking, "How is the world treating you?" I mumbled some response or other to the effect that things were going OK. Then he asked me, "And how are you treating the world?"

I was quite taken aback. It was the last question I was expecting. It was clear he didn't mean in a general way. He wasn't making pleasant conversation. He meant right there, on the retreat, that day, in what may have seemed to me at the time like little, even trivial ways. I thought I was more or less leaving "the world" in going on this retreat, but his comment drove home to me that there is no leaving the world, and that how I was relating to it in any and every moment, even in this artificially simplified environment, was important, in fact critical to my ultimate purpose in being there. I realized in that moment that I had a lot to learn about why I was even there in the first place, what meditation was really all about, and underlying it all, what I was really doing with my life.

Over the years, I gradually came to see the obvious, that the two questions are actually different sides of the same coin. For we are in intimate relationship with the world in all our moments. The give-and-take of that relationality is continually shaping our lives. It also shapes and defines the very world in which we live and in which our experiences unfold. Much of the time, we see these two aspects of life, how the world is treating me and how I am treating the world, as independent. Have you noticed how easily we can get caught up in thinking of ourselves as players on an inert stage, as if the world were only "out there" and not also "in here"? Have you noticed that we often act as if there were a significant separation between out there and in here, when our experience tells us that it is the thinnest of membranes, really no separation at all? Even if we sense the intimate relationship between outer and inner, still, we can be fairly insensitive to the ways our lives actually impinge upon and shape the world and the ways in which the world shapes our lives in a symbiotic dance of reciprocity and interdependence on every level, from intimacy with our own bodies and minds and what they are going through, to how we are relating to our family members; from our buying habits to what we think of the news we watch or don't watch on TV, to how we act or don't act within the larger world of the body politic.

That insensitivity is particularly onerous, even destructive, when we attempt, as we so often do, to force things to be a certain way, "my way," without regard for the potential violence, even on the tiniest but still significant scale, that such a break in the rhythm of things carries with it. Sooner or later, such forcing denies the reciprocity, the beauty of the give-and-take and the complexity of the dance itself; we wind up stepping, wittingly or unwittingly, on a lot of toes. Such insensitivity, such out-of-touchness, isolates us from our own possibilities. In refusing to acknowledge how things actually are in any moment, perhaps because we don't want them to be that way, and in attempting to compel a situation or a relationship to be the way we want it to be out of fear that otherwise we may not get our needs met, we are forgetting that most of the time we hardly know what our own way really is; we only think we do. And we forget that this dance is one of extraordinary complexity as well as simplicity, and that new and interesting things happen when we do not collapse in the presence of our fears, and instead stop imposing and start living our truth, well beyond our limited ability to assert tight control over anything for very long.

As individuals and as a species, we can no longer afford to ignore this fundamental characteristic of our reciprocity and interconnectedness, nor can we ignore how interesting new possibilities emerge out of our yearnings and our intentions when we are, each in our own way, actually true to them, however mysterious or opaque they may at times feel to us. Through our sciences, through our philosophies, our histories, and our spiritual traditions, we have come to see that our health and well-being as individuals, our happiness, and actually even the continuity of the germ line, that life stream that we are only a momentary bubble in, that way in which we are the life-givers and world-builders for our future generations, depend on how we choose to live our own lives while we have them to live.

At the same time, as a culture, we have come to see that the very Earth on which we live, to say nothing of the well-being of its creatures and its cultures, depends in huge measure on those same choices, writ large through our collective behavior as social beings.

To take just one example, which by now pretty much everybody knows about and honors, with a few notable exceptions, global temperatures can be accurately charted back at least 400,000 years and can be shown to fluctuate between extremes of hot and cold. We are in a relatively warm period, until recently not any warmer than any of the other warm eras Earth has experienced. In 2002, I was staggered to learn in a meeting between the Dalai Lama and a group of scientists that in the previous 44 years, atmospheric CO_2 levels shot up by 18 percent, to a higher level than in the past 160,000 years, as measured by carbon dioxide in snow cores in Antarctica. And the level is continuing to rise at an ever-increasing rate.* Now 2015, 2016, and 2017 appear to be the warmest years on record.

The dramatic and alarming recent increase in atmospheric CO_2 is entirely due to the activity of human beings. If unchecked, the Intergovernmental Panel on Climate Change predicts that levels of atmospheric CO_2 will double by 2100 and as a result, the average global temperature may rise dramatically. One consequence, as we all know, is that there is already open water at the North Pole in summer, ice is melting at both poles, and glaciers worldwide are rapidly disappearing. The potential consequences in terms of triggering chaotic fluctuations destabilizing the climate worldwide are sobering, if not terrifying, and we are seeing the results of that destabilization in the increasing severity of storms and their impact on our cities. While intrinsically unpredictable, the consequences include a possible dramatic rise in sea level in a relatively short period of time, and the flooding of all coastal habitations and cities worldwide. Imagine Manhattan if the ocean rises fifty feet. Think of Bangladesh, Puerto Rico, and all the coastal countries, cities, and islands where sea-level rise and more severe weather are already being felt.

We could say that these changes in temperature and weather patterns are one symptom, and only one among many, of a kind of autoimmune disease of the Earth, in that one aspect of human activity is seriously undermining the overall dynamic balance of the body of

---

* Steven Chu, Stanford University, Nobel laureate in physics, Mind and Life Institute, Dialogue X, Dharamsala, India, October 2002.

the earth as a whole. Do we know? Do we care? Is it somebody else's problem? "Their" problem, whoever "they" are...scientists, governments, politicians, utility companies, the auto industry? Is it possible, if we are really all part of one body, to collectively come to our senses on this issue and restore some kind of dynamical balance? Can we do that for any of the other ways in which our activity as a species threatens our very lives and the lives of generations to come, and, in fact, the lives of many other species as well?

To my mind, it is past time for us to pay attention to what we already know or sense, not just in the outer world of our relationships with others and with our surroundings, but in the interior world of our own thoughts and feelings, aspirations and fears, hopes and dreams. All of us, no matter who we are or where we live, have certain things in common. For the most part, we share the desire to live our lives in peace, to pursue our private yearnings and creative impulses, to contribute in meaningful ways to a larger purpose, to fit in and belong and be valued for who we are, to flourish as individuals and as families, and as societies of purpose and of mutual regard, to live in individual dynamic balance, which is health, and in a collective dynamic balance, what used to be called the "commonweal," which honors our differences and optimizes our mutual creativity and the possibility for a future free from wanton harm and from that which threatens what is most vital to our well-being and our very being.

Such a collective dynamic balance, in my view, would feel a lot like heaven, or at least like being comfortably at home. It is what peace feels like, when we really have peace and know peace, inwardly and outwardly. It is what being healthy feels like. It is what genuine happiness feels like. It is like being at home in the deepest of ways. Isn't that somehow what we are all claiming we really want?

Ironically, such balance is already here at our fingertips at all times, in little ways that are not so little and have nothing to do with wishful thinking, rigid or authoritarian control, or utopias. Such balance is already here when we tune in to our own bodies and minds and to those forces that move us forward through the day and through the years, namely our motivation and our vision of what is worth living for and what needs undertaking. It is here in the small acts of kindness that happen between strangers and in families and even, in times of war, between supposed enemies. It is here every time we recycle our bottles and newspapers, or think to conserve water, or act with others to care for our neighborhood or protect our dwindling wilderness areas and other species with whom we share this planet.

If we are suffering from an auto-immune disease of our very planet, and if the cause of that auto-immune disease stems from the activity and the mind states of human beings, then we might do well to consider what we might learn from the leading edge of modern medicine about the most effective approaches to such conditions. It turns out that in the past forty years, medicine has come to know, from a remarkable blossoming of research and clinical practices in the field variously known as mind/body medicine, behavioral medicine, psychosomatic medicine, and integrative medicine, that the mysterious, dynamic balance we call "health" involves both the body and the mind (to use our awkward and artificial way of speaking that bizarrely splits them from each other), and can be enhanced by specific qualities of attention that can be sustaining, restorative, and healing. It turns out that we all have, lying deep within us, in our hearts and in our very bones, a capacity for a dynamic, vital, sustaining inner peacefulness and well-being, and for a huge, innate, multifaceted intelligence that goes way beyond the merely conceptual. When we mobilize and refine that capacity and put it to use, we are much healthier physically, emotionally, and spiritually. And much happier. Even our thinking becomes clearer, and we are less plagued by storms in the mind.

This capacity for paying attention and for intelligent action can be cultivated, nurtured, and refined beyond our wildest dreams if we have the motivation to do so. Sadly, as individuals, that motivation often comes only when we have already experienced a life-threatening disease or a severe shock to the system that may leave us in tremendous pain in both soma and psyche. It may only come, as it does for so many of our patients taking the MBSR program in the Stress Reduction Clinic, once we are rudely awakened to the fact that no matter how remarkable our technological medicine, it has gross limitations that make complete cures a rarity, treatment often merely a rear-guard action to maintain the status quo, if there is any effective treatment at all, and even diagnosis of what is wrong an inexact and too often woefully inadequate science.

Without exaggeration, it is fair to say that new developments in medicine, neuroscience, and epigenetics, as noted in the Foreword, are showing that it is possible for individuals to mobilize deep innate resources we all seem to share by virtue of being human, resources for learning, for growing, for healing, and for transformation that are available to us across the entire life span. These capacities are folded into our chromosomes, our genes and genome, our brains, our bodies, our minds, and into our relationships with each other and with the world. We gain access to them starting from wherever we are, which is always here, and in the only moment we ever have, which is always now. We all have the potential for healing and transformation no matter what the situation we find ourselves in, of long duration or recently appearing, whether we see it as "good," "bad," or "ugly," hopeless or hopeful, whether we see the causes as internal or external. These inner resources are our birthright. They are available to us across our entire life span because they are not in any way separate from us. It is in our very nature as a species to learn and grow and heal and move toward greater wisdom in our ways of seeing and in our actions, and toward greater compassion for ourselves and others.

But still, these capacities need to be uncovered, developed, and put to use. Doing so is the challenge of our life's time, that is, a chance to make the most of the moments that we have. As a rule, our moments are easily missed or filled up with stuff, wanted and unwanted. But it is equally easy to realize that, in the unfolding of our lives, we actually have nothing but moments in which to live, and it is a gift to actually be present for them, and that interesting things start to happen when we are.

This challenge of a life's time, to choose to cultivate these capacities for learning, growing, healing, and transformation right in the midst of our moments, is also the adventure of a lifetime. It begins a journey toward realizing who we really are and living our lives as if they really mattered. And they do—more than we think. More than we can possibly think, and not merely for our own enjoyment or accomplishment, although our own joy and feelings of well-being and accomplishment are bound to blossom, all the same.

This journey toward greater health and sanity is catalyzed by mobilizing and developing resources we all already have. And the most important one is our capacity for paying attention, in particular to those aspects of our lives that we have not been according very much attention to, that we might say we have been ignoring, seemingly forever.

Paying attention refines and nurtures intimacy with awareness, that feature of our being that along with language, distinguishes the potential of our species for learning and for transformation, both individual and collective. We grow and change and learn and become aware through the direct apprehending of things through our five senses, coupled with our powers of mind, which Buddhists see as a sense in its own right. We are capable of perceiving that any one aspect of experience exists within an infinite web of interrelationships, some of which are critically important to our immediate or long-term well-being. True, we might not see many of those relationships right away. They may for now be more or less hidden dimensions within the fabric of our lives, yet to be discovered. Even so, these hidden dimensions, or what we might call *new degrees of freedom*, are potentially available to us, and will gradually reveal themselves to us as we continue to cultivate and dwell in our capacity for conscious awareness by attending intentionally with both awe and tenderness to the staggeringly complex yet fundamentally ordered universe, world, nation, geography, social terrain, family, mind, and body within which we locate and orient ourselves, all of which, at every level, is continually fluxing and changing, whether we know it or not, whether we like it or not, and thereby providing us with countless unexpected challenges and opportunities to wake up and to see more clearly, and thus to grow and to move toward greater wisdom in our actions, and toward quelling the tortured suffering of our tumultuous minds, habitually so far from home, so far from quiet and rest.

This journey toward health and sanity is nothing less than an invitation to wake up to the fullness of our lives while we actually have them to live, rather than only, if ever, on our deathbeds, which Henry David Thoreau warned against so eloquently in *Walden* when he wrote:

> I went to the woods because I wished to live deliberately, to front only the essential facts of life and see if I could not learn what it had to teach and not, when I came to die, discover that I had not lived.

Dying without actually fully living, without waking up to our lives while we have the chance, is an ongoing and significant risk for all of us, given the automaticity of our habits and the relentless pace at which events unfold in this era, far greater than in his, and the mindlessness that tends to pervade our relationships to what may be most important for us but, at the same time, least apparent in our lives.

But as Thoreau himself counseled, it is possible for us to learn to ground ourselves in our inborn capacity for wise and openhearted attention. He pointed out that it is both possible and highly desirable to first taste and then inhabit a vast and spacious awareness of both heart and mind. When properly cultivated, such awareness can discern, embrace, transcend and free us from the veils and limitations of our routinized thought patterns, our routinized senses, and routinized relationships, and from the frequently turbulent and destructive mind states and emotions that accompany them. Such habits are invariably conditioned by the past, not only through our genetic inheritance, but through our experiences of trauma, fear, lack of trust and safety, feelings of unworthiness from not having been seen and honored for who we were, or from long-standing resentment for past slights, injustices, or outright and overwhelming harm. Nevertheless, they are habits that narrow our view, distort our understanding, and, if unattended, prevent our growing and our healing.

To come to our senses, both literally and metaphorically, on the big scale as a species and on the smaller scale as a single human being, we first need to return to the body, the locus within which the biological senses and what we call the mind arise. The body is a place we mostly ignore; we may barely inhabit it at all, never mind attending to and honoring it. Our own body is, strangely, a landscape that is simultaneously both familiar and remarkably unfamiliar to us. It is a domain we might at times fear, or even loathe, depending on our past and what we have faced or fear we might. At other times, it may be something we are wholly seduced by, obsessed with the body's size, its shape, its weight, or look, at risk for falling into unconscious but seemingly endless self-preoccupation and narcissism.

At the level of the individual person, we know from many studies in the field of mind/body medicine in the past forty years that it is possible to come to some degree of peace within the body and mind and so find greater health, well-being, happiness, and clarity, even in the midst of great challenges and difficulties. Many thousands of people have already embarked on this journey through MBSR and have reported and continue to report remarkable benefits for themselves and for others with whom they share their lives and work. We have come to see that paying attention in such a way, and thereby tapping into those hidden dimensions and new degrees of freedom, is not a path for the select few. Anybody can embark on such a path and find great benefit and comfort in it.

Coming to our senses is the work of no time at all, only of being present and awake here and now. It is also, paradoxically, a lifetime's engagement. You could say we take it on "for life," in every sense of that phrase.

The first step on the adventure involved in coming to our senses on any and every level is the cultivation of intimacy with awareness itself. *Mindfulness* is synonymous with awareness. My operational definition of mindfulness is that it is "the awareness that arises from paying attention on purpose, in the present moment, and nonjudgmentally." If you need a reason for doing so, we could add "in the service of wisdom, self-understanding, and recognizing our intrinsic interconnectedness with others and with the world, and thus, also in the service of kindness and compassion." Mindfulness is intrinsically ethical, when one understands what "non-judgmental" really means.* It certainly doesn't mean that you won't have judgments—you will have plenty of those. It is an invitation to suspend the judging as best you can and simply recognize it when it arises, and not judge the judging.

Our capacity for awareness and for self-knowing could be said to be the final common pathway of what makes us human. We gain access to the power and wisdom of our own capacity for awareness though cultivating mindfulness. And mindfulness can be cultivated, developed, and refined, carefully and systematically, as a practice, as a way of being through *mindfulness meditation*.

The practice of mindfulness has been spreading rapidly around the world and into the mainstream of Western culture over the past forty years, thanks in large part to an ever-increasing number of scientific and medical studies of its various effects, and a consequent explosion of

---

* It does not eschew clarity and discernment, nor human values such as kindness and compassion.

interest in many different domains, including K–12 education, higher education, business, sports, criminal justice, the military, and government, to say nothing of psychology and psychotherapy.

There is nothing weird or out of the ordinary about meditating or meditation. It boils down to simply paying attention in your life as if it really really mattered—because it does, and more than you think. It might also help to keep in mind that while it is really nothing out of the ordinary, nothing particularly special, mindfulness is at the same time extraordinarily special and utterly transformative in ways that are impossible to imagine, although that won't stop us from trying.

When cultivated and refined, mindfulness can function to beneficial effect on virtually every level of human experience, from the individual to the corporate, the societal, the political, and the global. But it does require that we be motivated to realize who we actually are and to live our lives as if they really mattered, not just for ourselves, but for others and for our world. And that is because when we wake up, we realize that reality itself, and thus the world we inhabit, is characterized by deep interconnectedness. Nothing is really separate from anything else. And this interconnectedness becomes apparent the more we practice being awake and aware.

This adventure of a lifetime unfolds from whenever we take our first step. When we walk this path, as we will do together in this book and the other three volumes, we find that we are hardly alone in our efforts, nor are we alone or unique even in our life difficulties. For in taking up the practice of mindfulness, you are participating in what amounts to an ever-more robust global community of intentionality and exploration, one that ultimately includes all of us.

One more thing before we embark.

However much work we do on ourselves to learn and grow and heal what needs healing through the cultivation of mindfulness, it is not possible to be entirely healthy in a world that is profoundly unhealthy in some ways, and where it is apparent how much suffering and anguish there is in the world, both for those near and dear to us, and also for those unknown to us, whether around the corner or around the world. Being in reciprocal relationship to everything makes the suffering of others our suffering, whether or not we sometimes turn away from it because it is so painful to bear. Rather than being a problem, however, other people's suffering can be a strong motivating factor for both inner and outer transformation in ourselves and in the world.

It would not be an exaggeration to say that the world itself is suffering from a serious and progressive disease. A look back at history, anywhere and at any time, or just being alive now, plainly reveals that our world is subject to convulsive spasms of madness, periods of what looks like collective insanity, the ascendancy of narrow-mindedness and fundamentalism, times in which great misery and confusion and centrifugal forces pervade the status quo. These eruptions are the opposite of wisdom and balance. They tend to be compounded by a parochial arrogance usually devoted to self-aggrandizement and frank exploitation of others, inevitably associated with agendas of ideological, political, cultural, religious, or corporate hegemony, even as they are couched in a language of humanism, economic development, globalism, and the all-seductive lure of narrowly conceived views of material "progress" and Western-style democracy. These forces often carry the hidden expense of cultural or environmental homogenization and degradation, and the gross abrogation of human rights, all of which feel like they add up to an outright disease. The pendulum swings seem to be coming faster and faster, so there is little time we can actually point to when we are in between such convulsive spasms and actually feeling at ease and benefiting from a pervading peacefulness.

We know that the twentieth century saw more organized killing in the name of peace and tranquility and the end of war than all centuries past combined, the vast majority of it erupting, ironically perhaps, in the great centers of learning and magnificent culture that are Europe and the Far East. And the twenty-first century is following on apace, if in a different but equally, if not more, disturbing mode. Whoever the protagonists, and whatever the rhetoric and the particular issues of contention, wars, including covert wars and wars against terror, are always put forth in the name of the highest and most compelling of purposes and principles by all sides. They always lead to murderous bloodletting that in the end, even when apparently unavoidable, harms both victims and perpetrators. And they are always caused by disturbances in the human mind. Engaging in harming others to resolve disputes that could be better resolved in other, more imaginative ways, also blinds us to the ways in which war and violence are themselves symptoms of the auto-immune disease from which our species seems to uniquely and collectively suffer. It blinds us as well to other ways available to us to restore harmony and balance when they are disrupted by very real, very dangerous, even virulent forces that we may unwittingly be helping to feed and expand, even as we abhor them and vigorously resist and combat them.

What is more, "winning" a war nowadays is a far different challenge than winning the peace in a war's aftermath, as America has had to face up to in Iraq and Afghanistan. For that, an entirely different order of thinking and awareness and planning is required, one that can only come from understanding ourselves better and coming to a more gracious understanding of others who may not aspire to what we hold to be most important, who have their own culture and customs and values, and who may, hard as it is sometimes for us to believe, perceive the same events quite differently from how we might be perceiving them. The United States actually accomplished this in a remarkably prescient manner through the compassionate genius and wisdom of the Marshall Plan in Europe after the Second World War.

All the same, we need continually to recognize the relativity of perception and the motivations that may both shape and derive from those perceptions, caught in restrictive loops that prevent a greater, more inclusive, and perhaps more accurate seeing. Given the condition of the world, perhaps it is time for us all to tap into a deeper dimension of human intelligence and commonality that underlies our different ways of seeing and knowing. This suggests that it may be profoundly unwise to focus solely on our own individual well-being and security, because our well-being and security are intimately interconnected with everything else in this ever-contracting world we inhabit. Coming to our senses involves cultivating an overarching awareness of all our senses, including our own minds *and their limitations,* including the temptation when we feel deeply insecure and have a lot of resources, to try to control as rigidly and as tightly as possible all variables in the external world, an impossible and ultimately depleting, intrinsically violent, and self-exhausting enterprise.

In the larger domain of the world's health, as in the case of our own life, because it is so basic, we will need to give primacy to awareness of the body, but in this case, it is the body politic, the "body" constituted of communities and corporations (the very word means body), nations and families of nations, all of which have their own corresponding ills, diseases, and mix of views, as well as profound resources for cultivating self-awareness and healing within their own traditions and cultures and, beyond them, in the confluence of many different cultures and traditions, one of the hallmarks of today's world.

An auto-immune disease is really the body's own self-sensing, surveillance, and security system, the immune system, gone amok, attacking its own cells and tissues, attacking itself. No body and no body politic can thrive for long under such conditions, with one part of itself warring on another, no matter how healthy and vibrant it may be in other ways. Nor can any country thrive for long in the world with a foreign policy defined to a large extent by allergic reaction, one manifestation of a disregulated immune system, nor on the excuse, true as it may be, that we are collectively suffering from severe post-traumatic stress following the September 11, 2001 attacks. That trauma was only compounded by the arising of ISIS and of global terrorism. The ascendency of currents of toxic and racist populism was not far behind. Such conditions only make it easier for either well-meaning or cynical leaders to exploit events for purposes that have little or nothing to do with healing or with true security or authentic democracy, for that matter.

As with an individual who is catapulted, however rudely and unexpectedly, onto the road to greater health and well-being by a nonlethal heart attack or some other untoward and unexpected diagnosis, a shock to the system, horrific as it may be, can, if held and understood with care and attention, be the occasion of a wake-up call to mobilize the deep and powerful resources that are at our disposal for healing and for redirecting our energies and priorities, resources that we may have too long neglected or even forgotten we possess, even as we respond mindfully and forcefully to ensure our safety and well-being.

Such healing of the greater world is the work of many generations. It has already begun in many places as we realize the enormity of the risks we face by not paying attention to the moribund condition of the patient, which is the world; by not paying attention to the history of the patient, which is life on this planet and, in particular, human life, since its activities are now shaping the destiny of all beings on Earth for lifetimes to come; by not paying attention to the auto-immune diagnosis that is staring us in the face but which we are finding it difficult to accept; and by not paying attention to the potential for treatment that involves a widespread embracing of what is deepest and best in our own nature as living and therefore sensing beings, while there is still time to do so.

Healing our world will involve learning, however tentatively, to put our multiple intelligences to work in the service of life, liberty, and the pursuit of real happiness, for ourselves, and for generations of beings to come. Not just for Americans and Westerners either, but for all inhabitants of this planet, whatever continent or island we reside on. And not just for human beings, but for all beings in the natural, more-than-human world, what Buddhists often refer to as *sentient beings.*

For sentience, when all is said and done, is the key to coming to our senses and waking up to the possible. Without awareness, without learning how to use, refine, and inhabit our consciousness, our genetic capacity for clear seeing and selfless action, both within ourselves as individuals and within our institutions—including businesses, the House and the Senate, the White House, seats of government, and larger gatherings of nations such as the United Nations and the European Union—we are dooming ourselves to the auto-immune disease of our own unawareness, from which stem endless rounds of illusion, delusion, greed, fear, cruelty, self-deception, and ultimately, wanton destruction and death. It is humankind, the human species itself, that is the auto-immune disease of planet Earth. We are the disease agent and also its first victim. But that is not the end of the story by any means. At least not yet. Not now.

For as long as we are breathing, there is still time to choose life, and to reflect on what such a choice is asking of us. This choice is a nitty-gritty, moment-to-moment one, not some colossal or intimidating abstraction. It is very close to the substance and substrate of our lives unfolding in whatever ways they do, inwardly in our thoughts and feelings, and outwardly in our words and deeds moment by moment by moment.

The world needs all its flowers, just as they are, and even though they bloom for only the briefest of moments, which we call a lifetime. It is our job to find out one by one and collectively what kind of flowers we are, and to share our unique beauty with the world in the precious time that we have, and to leave our children and grandchildren a legacy of wisdom and compassion embodied in the way we live, in our institutions, and in our honoring of our interconnectedness, at home and around the world. Why not risk standing firmly for sanity in our lives and in our world, the inner and the outer a reflection of each other and of our genius as a species?

The creative and imaginative efforts and actions of every one of us count, and nothing less than the health of the world hangs in the balance. We could say that the world is literally and metaphorically dying for us as a species to come to our senses, and now is the time. Now is the time for us to wake up to the fullness of our beauty, to get on with and amplify the work of healing ourselves, our societies, and the planet, building on everything worthy that has come before and that is flowering now. No intention is too small and no effort insignificant. Every step along the way counts. And, as you will see, every single one of us counts.

As described in the Foreword, this book is now the first of four volumes, each with a Part 1 and a Part 2. Throughout all four books, I have woven here and there stories of my own personal experience. This is with the aim of giving the reader a feeling sense of the paradox of how personal and particular meditation practice is on the one hand, and at the same time, how impersonal and universal it is on the other, beyond any self-involved story line of "my" experience, "my" life that the mind's persistent selfing habit may cook up; a feeling sense of how important it is to take one's experience seriously but not personally, and with a healthy dose of lightheartedness and humor, especially in the face of the colossal suffering we are immersed in by virtue of being human, and in light of the ultimate evanescence of those distorting lenses called our opinions and our views that we so often cling to in trying desperately to make sense of the world and of ourselves.

In Part 1 of this volume, we will explore what meditation is and isn't, and what is involved in the cultivation of mindfulness. Part 2 examines the root sources of our suffering and "dis-ease" and how paying attention on purpose and non-judgmentally is itself liberating, how mindfulness has been integrated into medicine, and how it reveals new dimensions of our minds and hearts that can be profoundly restorative and transforming.

In Book 2 (*Falling Awake*), Part 1 explores the "sensescapes" of our lives and how greater awareness of the senses feeds our well-being and enriches our lives and our ways of knowing and being in the world and within our own interiority. Part 2 gives the reader detailed instructions for the cultivating of mindfulness through the various senses, making use of a range of formal meditation practices, and thus gives a taste of their exquisite richness, available to us in every moment.

In Book 3 (*The Healing Power of Mindfulness*), Part 1 explores how the cultivation of mindfulness can lead to healing and to greater happiness through what I call an "orthogonal rotation in consciousness" in the ways we apprehend and then act in the world.* Part 2 expands on the cultivation of mindfulness and gives a range of examples of how it can affect various aspects of our daily lives, everything from experiencing the place you are in to watching or not watching the Super Bowl, to "dying before we die."

In Book 4 (*Mindfulness for All*), Part 1 looks at the world of politics and the stress of the world from the perspective of mind/body medicine, and suggests some ways in which mindfulness may help transform and further the health of the body politic and of the world. Part 2 frames our lives and the challenges facing us in the present moment in the greater context and perspective of the species itself and our evolution on the planet, and reveals the hidden dimensions of the possible that allow us to live our lives from moment to moment and from day to day as if they really mattered.

---

* No need to be intimidated by the big word. It just means "at ninety degrees" in relationship to the coordinate system being used. Think of it as describing a new dimension beyond the conventional ones we are familiar with to give us a new perspective on the whole, based on that greater dimensionality.

As noted earlier, there is a progression through the four volumes, from the "What" and the "Why" of mindfulness to the "How" of cultivating it in our own lives, to the reasons we might be motivated to do so—in other words, the "Promise" of mindfulness—to its Realization in how we actually lead our lives from moment to moment. I hope you find them nourishing.

PART 1

MEDITATION

———

It's Not What You Think

*The range of what we think and do
is limited by what we fail to notice.*

R. D. LAING

*There is that in me . . . I do not know what it is . . . but I know
it is in me.*

WALT WHITMAN

MEDITATION IS NOT FOR THE FAINT-HEARTED

It is difficult to speak of the timeless beauty and richness of the present moment when things are moving so fast. But the faster things move, the more important it is for us to dip into or even inhabit the timeless. Otherwise, we can lose touch with dimensions of our humanity that make all the difference between happiness and misery, between wisdom and folly, between well-being and the erosive turmoil in the mind, in the body, and in the world that we will be referring to as "dis-ease." Because our discontent truly is a disease, even when it does not appear as such. Sometimes we colloquially refer to those kinds of feelings and conditions, to that "dis-ease" we feel so much of the time, as "stress." It is usually painful. It weighs on us. And it always carries a feeling of underlying dissatisfaction.

In 1979 I started a Stress Reduction Clinic at the University of Massachusetts Medical Center in Worcester, Massachusetts. Thinking back to that era, almost forty years ago, I ask myself, "What stress?" so much has our world changed since then, so much has the pace of life increased and the vagaries and dangers of the world come to our doorstep as never before. If looking squarely at our personal situation and circumstances and finding novel and imaginative ways to work with them in the service of health and healing was important forty years ago, it is infinitely more important and urgent now, inhabiting as we do a world that has been thrown into heightened chaos and speed in the unfolding of events, even as it has become far more interconnected and smaller.

In such an exponentially accelerating and ever more disruptive era, it is more important and urgent than ever for us to learn to inhabit the timeless and draw upon it for solace and clear seeing. That has been, from the start, the very core of the curriculum of our Stress Reduction Clinic, what is now known as MBSR (mindfulness-based stress reduction). I am not speaking of some distant future in which, after years of striving, you would finally attain something, taste the timeless beauty of meditative awareness and all it offers, and ultimately lead a more effective and satisfying and peaceful life in some fantasy future that may or may not ever arrive. I am speaking of accessing the timeless in this very moment—because it is always right under our noses, so to speak—and in so doing, to gain access to those dimensions of possibility that are presently hidden from us because we refuse to be present, because we are seduced, entrained, mesmerized, or frightened into the future and the past, carried along in the stream of events and the weather patterns of our own reactions and numbness, attending to, if not obsessing about what we often unthinkingly dub "urgent," while losing touch at the same time with what is actually important, supremely important, in fact vital for our own well-being, for our sanity, and for our very survival. We have made absorption in the future and in the past such an overriding habit that, much of the time, we have no awareness of the present moment at all. As a consequence, we may feel we have very little, if any, control over the ups and downs of our own lives and of our own minds.

The opening sentence of the brochure in which we described the mindfulness retreats and training programs that our institute, the Center for Mindfulness in Medicine, Health Care, and Society (the CFM for short), offered for many years to business leaders read: "Meditation is not for the faint-hearted nor for those who routinely avoid the whispered longings of their own hearts." That sentence was very much there on purpose. Its aim was to immediately discourage from attending those who were not yet ready for the timeless, who wouldn't understand or even make enough room in their minds or hearts to give such an experience or understanding a chance.

If they had come to one of those five-day programs, chances are they would have found themselves fighting with their own mind the entire time, thinking the meditation practice was nonsense, pure torture, boring in the extreme, a waste of time. Chances are they would have been so caught up in their resisting and objecting that they might never have found a way to settle into the precious and preciously brief moments we have when we are able to get together to explore our actual moment-by-moment experience in such ways.

And if people did show up at these retreats, we could assume that it was either because of that sentence or in spite of it. Either way, or so our strategizing went, there would be an implicit if not intrepid willingness on the part of those who did show up to explore the interior landscape of the mind and body, and the realm of what the ancient Chinese Taoists and Chan masters called *non-doing*, the domain of true meditation, in which it looks as though nothing or nothing much is happening or being done, but at the same time, nothing important is left undone—and as a consequence, that mysterious energy of an open, aware non-doing can manifest in the world of doing in remarkable ways.

Of course we all mostly avoid the whispered longings of our own hearts as we are carried along in the stream of life's doings, especially as our attention is pulled in so many different directions and we become more and more distracted. And I am certainly not suggesting that meditation is always easy or pleasant. It is simple, but it certainly isn't always easy. It is not easy to string even a few moments together in which to practice formally on a regular basis in a busy life, never mind remembering that mindfulness is available to us, you might say "informally," in any and every unfolding moment of our lives. But sometimes we can no longer ignore those intimations from our own hearts. And sometimes, somehow, we find ourselves pulled to show up in places we ordinarily wouldn't, mysteriously drawn to where we might have lived for a time as a child, or to the wilderness, or to a meditation retreat, or to a book or a class or to a conversation that might offer that long-ignored side of ourselves a chance to open to the sunlight, to be seen and heard and felt and known and inhabited by ourselves, by our own heart's lifelong longing to meet itself.

The adventure that the universe of mindfulness offers is one possible avenue into dimensions of your being that may have perhaps gone ignored and unattended or denied for too long. Mindfulness, as we will see, has a rich and textured capacity to influence the unfolding of our lives. By the same token, it has an equal capacity to influence the larger world within which we are seamlessly embedded, including our family, our work, the society as a whole and how we see ourselves as a people, what I am calling the body politic, and the body of the world, of all of us together on this planet. And all this can come about through your own experience of the practice of mindfulness by virtue of that very embeddedness and the reciprocal relationships between inner and outer, and between being and doing.

For there is no question that we are seamlessly embedded in the web of life itself and within the web of what we might call mind, an invisible intangible essence that allows for sentience and conscious-ness and the potential for awareness itself to transform ignorance into wisdom and discord into reconciliation and accord. Awareness offers a safe haven in which to restore ourselves and rest in a vital and dynamic harmony, tranquility, creativity, and joyfulness now, not in some far-off hoped-for future time when things are "better" or we have gotten things under control, or have "improved" ourselves. Strange as it may sound, our capacity for mindfulness allows us to taste and embody that which we most deeply desire, that which most eludes us and which is, curiously, always ever so close, a greater stabil-ity and peace of mind and all that accompanies it, in any and every moment available to us.

In microcosm, peace is no farther than this very moment. In macrocosm, peace is something almost all of us collectively aspire to in one way or another, especially if it is accompanied by justice, and recognition of an intrinsic diversity within our larger wholeness, and of everybody's innate humanity and rights. Peace is something that we can bring about if we can actually learn to wake up a bit more as individuals and a lot more as a species; if we can learn to be fully what we actually already are; to reside in the inherent potential of what is possible for us, being human. As the adage goes, "There is no way to peace; peace is the way." It is so for the outer landscape of the world. It is so for the inner landscape of the heart. And these are, in a profound way, not really two.

Because mindfulness, which can be thought of as an openhearted, moment-to-moment, non-judgmental awareness, is optimally cultivated through meditation rather than just through merely thinking about it and philosophizing, and because its most elaborate and complete articulation comes from the Buddhist tradition, in which mindfulness is often described as *the heart of Buddhist meditation*, I have chosen to say some things here and there as we go along about Buddhism and its relationship to the practice of mindfulness. I do this so that we might reap some understanding and some benefit from what this extraordinary tradition offers the world at this moment in history, based on its incubation on our planet in many different cultures over the past twenty-six hundred years.

The way I see it, Buddhism itself is not the point. You might think of the Buddha as a genius of his age, a great scientist, at least as towering a figure as Darwin or Einstein, who, as the Buddhist scholar Alan Wallace likes to put it, had no instruments other than his own mind at his disposal and who sought to look deeply into the nature of birth and death and the seeming inevitability of suffering. In order to pursue his investigations, he first had to understand, develop, refine, and learn to calibrate and stabilize the instrument he was using for this purpose, namely his own mind, in the same way that laboratory scientists today have to continually develop, refine, calibrate, and stabilize the instruments that they employ to extend their senses—whether we are talking about giant optical or radio telescopes, electron microscopes, functional magnetic resonance imaging (fMRI) scanners, or positron-emission tomography (PET) scanners—in the service of looking deeply into and exploring the nature of the universe and the vast array of interconnected phenomena that unfold within it, whether it be in the domain of physics and physical phenomena, chemistry, biology, psychology, or any other field of inquiry.

To meet this challenge, the Buddha and those who followed in his footsteps took on exploring deep questions about the nature of the mind itself and about the nature of life. Their efforts at self-observation led to remarkable discoveries. They succeeded in accurately mapping a territory that is quintessentially human, having to do with aspects of the mind that we all have in common, independent of our particular thoughts, beliefs, and cultures. Both the methods they used and the fruits of those investigations are universal, and have nothing to do with any isms, ideologies, religiosities, or belief systems. These discoveries are more akin to medical and scientific understandings, frameworks that can be examined by anybody anywhere, and put to the test independently for oneself, which is what the Buddha suggested to his followers from the very beginning.

Because I practice and teach mindfulness, I have the recurring experience that people frequently make the assumption that I am a Buddhist. When asked, I usually respond that I am not a Buddhist (although I do practice on retreat with Buddhist teachers from time to time and have great respect and love for different Buddhist traditions and practices), but I am a student of Buddhist meditation, and a devoted one, not because I am devoted to Buddhism per se, but because I have found its core teachings and practices to be so profound and so universally applicable, illuminating, and healing,* I have found this to be the case in my own life over the past fifty-plus years of ongoing practice, and I have found it to be the case as well in the lives of many others with whom I have had the privilege of working and practicing through the Center for Mindfulness and its global network of MBSR teachers. And I continue to be deeply touched and inspired by those teachers and nonteachers alike—Easterners and Westerners, who embody the wisdom and compassion inherent in these teachings and practices in their own lives.

For me, mindfulness practice is really a love affair, a love affair with what is most fundamental in life, a love affair with what is so, with what we might call truth, which for me includes beauty, the unknown, and the possible, how things actually are, all embedded here, in this very moment—for it is all already here—and at the same time, everywhere, because here can be anywhere at all. Mindfulness is also always now, because as we have already touched on, and as we will touch on many times again, for us there simply is no other time.

Here and now, everywhere and always, gives us a lot of room for working together, that is, if you are interested and willing to roll up your sleeves and do the work of the timeless, the work of non-doing, the work of awareness embodied in your own life as it is always unfolding moment by moment. It is indeed the work of no time at all, and the work of a lifetime.

No one culture and no one art form has a monopoly on either truth or beauty, writ either large or small. But for the particular exploration we will be undertaking together in these pages and in our lives, I find it is both useful and illuminating to draw upon the work of those special people on our planet who devote themselves to the language

---

* See for example, the recent and improbable bestseller, *Why Buddhism Is True*, by Robert Wright, 2017.

of the mind and heart that we call poetry. Our greatest poets engage in deep interior explorations of the mind and of words and of the intimate relationship between inner and outer landscapes, just as do the greatest yogis and teachers in the meditative traditions. In fact, it is not uncommon in the meditative traditions for moments of illumination and insight to be expressed through poetry. Both yogis and poets are intrepid explorers of what is so, and articulate guardians of the possible.

The lenses that great poetry holds up for us, as with all authentic art, have the potential to enhance our seeing, and even more importantly, our ability to feel the poignancy and relevance of our own situations, our own psyches, and our own lives, in ways that help us to understand where the meditation practice may be asking us to look and to see, what it is asking us to open to, and above all, what it is making possible for us to feel and to know. Poetry emanates from all the cultures and traditions of this planet. One might say our poets are the keepers of the conscience and the soul of our humanity, and have been through all the ages. They speak many aspects of a truth worth attending to and contemplating. North American, Central American, South American, Chinese, Japanese, European, Turkish, Persian, Indian or African, Christian, Jewish, Islamic, Buddhist, Hindu or Jain, animist or classical, women and men, ancients and moderns, gay or straight, trans or queer, all might, under the right circumstances, when we are most open and available to ourselves, bestow a mysterious gift upon us worth exploring, savoring, and cherishing. They give us fresh lenses with which to see and come to know ourselves across the span of cultures and of time, offering something more fundamental, something more human than the expected or the already known. The view through such lenses may not always be comforting. At times, it might be downright disturbing and perturbing. And perhaps those are the poems that we most need to linger with because they reveal the ever-changing full spectrum of light and shadow that plays across the screens of our own minds, and moves within the subterranean currents of our own hearts. In their best moments poets articulate the inexpressible, and in such moments, by some mysterious grace bestowed by muse and heart, are transfigured into masters of words beyond words, the unspeakable wrought and fashioned and pointed to, brought to life in part by our own participation in them. Poems are animated when we come to them and let them come to us in that moment of reading or hearing when we hang with all our sensibilities and intelligences on every word, every event or moment evoked, every breath drawn to evoke it, every image invoked with vibrancy and art, carrying us beyond artifice, back to ourselves and what is actually so.

To that end, we will pause now and again on our journey together through the four of these books to bathe in these waters of clarity and of anguish and so be bathed by the ineluctable efforts of humanity yearning to know itself, reminding itself of what it does know, sometimes even succeeding, and in a deeply friendly and ultimately hugely generous and compassionate act, although hardly ever undertaken for that purpose, pointing out possible ways of deepening our living and our seeing and feeling, and perhaps thereby appreciating more—and even celebrating—who and what we are, and might become.

*

My heart rouses
> *thinking to bring you news*
>> *of something*
that concerns you
> *and concerns many men. Look at*
>> *what passes for the new.*
You will not find it there but in
> *despised poems.*
>> *It is difficult*
to get the new from poems
> *yet men die miserably every day*

for lack
of what is found there.

WILLIAM CARLOS WILLIAMS

*

Outside, the freezing desert night.
This other night grows warm, kindling.
Let the landscape be covered with thorny crust.
We have a soft garden in here.
The continents blasted,
cities and towns, everything
becomes a scorched, blackened ball.

The news we hear is full of grief for that future,
but the real news inside here
is there's no news at all.

RUMI
Translated by Coleman Barks with John Moyne

WITNESSING HIPPOCRATIC INTEGRITY

I am lying on the carpeted floor of the spacious and spanking new Faculty Conference Room at the UMass Medical Center with a group of about fifteen patients in the dwindling light of a late September afternoon in 1979. This is the first class in the first cycle of the Stress Reduction and Relaxation Program, later to become known as the Stress Reduction Clinic, or MBSR (for mindfulness-based stress reduction) Clinic that has just been launched here. I am midway through guiding us in an extended lying-down meditation known as the body scan. We are all lying on our backs on brand-new cloth-encased foam mats of various bright colors, clustered together at one end of the room so as better to hear my instructions.

In the middle of a long stretch of silence, the door to the room suddenly opens and a group of about thirty people in long white coats enters. In the lead is a tall and stately gentleman. He strides over to where I am lying and gazes first down upon me, stretched out on the floor in a black T-shirt and black karate pants, barefoot, then around the room, a quizzical and bemused look on his face.

He looks down at me again, and, after a long pause, finally says, "What is going on here?" I remain lying down, and so does the rest of the class, corpse-like on their colorful mats, their attention suspended somewhere between their feet, where we had started out, and the top of the head, where we were headed, with all the white coats silently looming in the shadows behind this commanding presence. "This is the hospital's new stress-reduction program," I reply, still lying there, wondering to myself what on Earth was going on. He responded, "Well, this is a special joint meeting of the surgical faculty with the faculty of all our affiliate hospitals, and we specifically had this conference room reserved for this purpose for some time."

At this point, I stand up. My head comes up to about his shoulder. I introduce myself and say, "I can't imagine how this conflict came about. I double-checked with the scheduling office to make sure we had the room reserved for our Wednesday afternoon classes for the next ten weeks for this time slot, from four to six p.m."

He looked me up and down, towering over me in his long white coat with his name embroidered in blue on the front: H. Brownell Wheeler, MD, Chief of Surgery. He had never seen me before, and had certainly not heard of this new program. We must have looked a sight, with our shoes and sox off, many in sweats and work-out clothes, lying on the floor of the faculty conference room. Here was one of the most powerful people in the medical center, with the clock ticking on his busy schedule and a special meeting to facilitate,* encountering something completely unexpected and on the face of it, bizarre in the extreme, led by someone with virtually no standing in the medical center.

He looked around one more time, at all the bodies on the floor, some by this time propped up on the elbows to take in what was going on. And then he asked one question.

"Are these our patients?" he inquired, gazing around at the bodies on the floor.

"Yes," I replied. "They are."

---

* I learned much later that this meeting was called to address and hopefully diffuse at least some of the friction that had arisen between the relatively new medical center and the local community hospitals over terminating the individual community hospital surgical residency programs and creating a single "integrated" UMass program, which had led to a good deal of resentment directed at UMass. So Dr. Wheeler had a lot riding on this meeting and it was important for him to hold it in this very inviting and congenial space.

"Then we will find someplace else to hold our meeting," he said, and he turned around and led the whole group out of the room.

I thanked him, closed the door behind them, and got back on the floor to resume our work.

That was my introduction to Brownie Wheeler. I knew in that moment that I was going to enjoy working at that medical center.

Years later, after Brownie and I had become friends, I reminded him of that episode, and told him how impressed I had been at his uncompromising respect for the hospital's patients. Characteristically, he didn't think it a big deal. There was just no compromising on the principle that patients come first, no matter what.

By that time, I knew that he himself practiced meditation and was deeply appreciative of the power of the mind-body connection and its potential to transform medicine. He was a staunch supporter of the Stress Reduction Clinic for more than two decades. Then, having stepped down as Chief of Surgery, he became a leader in the movement to bring dignity and kindness to the process of dying, before succumbing years later to Parkinson's disease. At the request of his daughter, we reconnected by phone, with me doing the talking for both of us, a few days before he died.

That he didn't use his power and authority to dominate the situation on that late afternoon in the prime of his life and of his power in the medical center left me knowing that I had just witnessed and become the beneficiary of something all-too-rare in our society: embodied wisdom and compassion. The respect he showed the patients on that day was exactly what the meditation practice we were doing when the door to the conference room opened was attempting to nourish: A deep and non-judging acceptance of ourselves and the cultivation of our own transformative and healing possibilities. Dr. Wheeler's gracious gesture that afternoon augured well for honoring the ancient Hippocratic principles of medicine, so sorely needed in this world in so many ways, in more than merely fine words. No fine words were uttered. And nothing was left unsaid.

Meditation Is Everywhere

Picture this: Medical patients meditating and doing yoga in hospitals and medical centers around the country and around the world at the urging of their doctors. Sometimes it is even the doctors who are doing the teaching. Sometimes doctors are taking the program and meditating shoulder to shoulder alongside the patients.

Andries Kroese, a prominent vascular surgeon in Oslo who had been practicing meditation for thirty years and attending vipassana* retreats in India periodically, came to California to participate in a seven-day retreat for health professionals wanting to train in MBSR. Shortly after returning home, he decided to cut back on his surgical practice and use the time he freed up to teach meditation to colleagues and patients in Scandinavia, a passion he had harbored for years. He then wrote a popular book about mindfulness-based stress reduction in Norwegian which became a best seller in Norway and Sweden. He is still at it more than a decade later.

Harold Nudelman, a surgeon from El Camino Hospital in Mountain View, California, called one day. He introduced himself as having melanoma, and said he feared he did not have long to live. He said he was familiar with meditation and had found it to be personally life-changing. After coming across my book *Full Catastrophe Living*, he recounted, he realized that we had already found a way to do what

---

* Mindfulness meditation in the Theravadan Buddhist tradition.

he had been dreaming of for quite some time, namely to bring meditation into mainstream medicine. He said he wanted to facilitate that happening in his hospital in whatever time he had left. A month later, he brought a team of doctors and administrators to visit us. Upon returning home, they set up an MBSR program led by a superb mindfulness teacher, Bob Stahl, who brought in other wonderful teachers as the program grew. It is still going more than twenty years later. Howard never bothered to tell me that he was the president of the board of a group seeking to build a mindfulness meditation retreat center in the Bay Area (which ultimately became the Spirit Rock Meditation Center in Woodacre, California). He died within a year of his visit. Brownie Wheeler, to whom I had introduced him during his group's visit with us, delivered the inaugural Howard Nudelman Memorial Lecture at El Camino Hospital later that year.

El Camino is now one of numerous hospitals, medical centers, and clinics in the San Francisco Bay area that are offering MBSR, including, at the time of writing, many within the Kaiser Permanente system in Northern California. Kaiser even offers mindfulness training for its physicians and staff as well as for its patients. MBSR programs are flourishing from Seattle to Miami, from Worcester, Massachusetts, where it began, to San Diego, California, from Whitehorse, Yukon Territory, to Vancouver, Calgary, Toronto, and Halifax, from Beijing and Shanghai to Hong Kong and Taiwan, from England and Wales to pretty much all of Europe, from Mexico to Colombia to Argentina. There are programs in Capetown, South Africa, and in Australia and New Zealand. There are long-standing MBSR programs at the medical centers of Duke, Stanford, the University of Wisconsin, the University of Virginia, Jefferson Medical College, and at other prominent medical centers across the country. Increasing numbers of scientists are now conducting clinical studies on the applications of mindfulness in both medicine and psychology. In the early 2000s, inspired by and modeled on MBSR, three cognitive therapists and researchers developed MBCT (mindfulness-based cognitive therapy). MBCT has been shown, through numerous clinical trials, to dramatically reduce the rate of relapse in people suffering with major depressive disorder. MBCT was also shown to be at least as effective as antidepressant therapy itself for preventing relapse. This program has generated an enormous amount of interest in clinical psychology and prompted new generations of psychologists and psychotherapists to take up the practice of mindfulness meditation in their own lives and apply it in their clinical work and research. (See the chapter titled "You Can't Get There From Here") in *The Healing Power of Mindfulness* (the third book in this series).

Forty years ago it was virtually inconceivable that meditation and yoga would find any legitimate role, no less widespread acceptance, in academic medical centers and hospitals. Now it is considered normal. It is certainly not thought of as alternative medicine. Rather it is just another element of the practice of good medicine. Increasingly, programs in mindfulness are now available for medical students and for hospital staff, both unfortunately under high stress.

There are even programs in some hospitals that teach meditation to patients in the bone marrow transplant unit, at the very high-tech, invasive end of the medical treatment spectrum. These were pioneered by my longtime colleague in the Stress Reduction Clinic, Elana Rosenbaum, who underwent a bone marrow transplant herself when she was diagnosed with lymphoma and so amazed the staff and physicians on the unit with the quality of her being, given that the complications she experienced following the treatment took her to death's door, that many wanted to take the program and learn to practice mindfulness for themselves and to offer it to their patients while they were on the unit. There are MBSR programs for inner-city residents and the homeless. There are MBSR programs in the United States taught entirely in Spanish. There are mindfulness programs for pain patients, for cancer patients, and for cardiac patients. Now there is MBCP (mindfulness-based Childbirth and Parenting), developed by MBSR teacher and midwife, Nancy Bardacke, for expectant parents, based at the Osher Center for Integrative Medicine at UCSF.

Many patients don't wait for their doctors to suggest MBSR and other mindfulness-based programs any more. These days, they ask for it, or just show up on their own.

Mindfulness meditation is also being taught in law firms and has at times been offered to law students at Yale, Columbia, Harvard, Missouri, Gainesville, and elsewhere. My colleague, Rhonda Magee, a professor of law at San Francisco University, has developed robust mindfulness-based courses for lawyers and law students that are also aimed at minimizing social-identity-based bias. A pioneering symposium on mindfulness and the law and alternative dispute resolution took place at Harvard Law School in 2002 and the papers presented were published in an issue of the *Harvard Negotiation Law Review* that same year. There is a whole movement now within the legal profession where lawyers themselves are teaching yoga and meditation in prominent law firms. One senior lawyer all dressed up in suit and tie was featured recently on the cover of the *Boston Globe Sunday Magazine* doing the tree pose, smiling—in bare feet—for an article on "The New (Kinder, Gentler) Lawyer."

What is going on?

As mentioned, business leaders and now, increasingly tech leaders attend rigorous five-day retreats that start at six o'clock each morning and go late into the evening. Their motivation: to change the world, and regulate their own stress levels, and to bring greater awareness to the life of business and the business of life. Many pioneering schools and school systems, such as in Flint, Michigan, are instituting mindfulness programs at the elementary, middle school, and high school levels. There are groups like Mindful Schools and Mindfulness in Schools, and Daniel Rechtshaffen's Mindful Education Online Training for teachers, all of whom are doing remarkable work and seeing profound results in both K–12 classroom teachers and their students. In the domain of sport, during Phil Jackson's era as coach of the Chicago Bulls, the team trained in and practiced mindfulness under the guidance of George Mumford, who headed our prison project at the Center for Mindfulness and also cofounded our inner-city MBSR clinic. When Jackson moved to Los Angeles to coach the Lakers, they too practiced mindfulness. Both teams were NBA champions, the Bulls six times (three with George), and the Lakers five times (all with George).* Now it is the champion Golden State Warriors who have adopted mindfulness as part of their approach to the game, encouraged by their head coach, Steve Kerr, who was exposed to it when he was on the championship Bulls teams. Prisons offer programs in meditation to inmates and staff alike, not only in this country, but in places like the UK and India.

One summer I had the occasion to co-lead, with the Alaskan fisherman, Zen practitioner, and now MBSR teacher Kurt Hoelting of Inside Passages, a meditation retreat for environmental activists that included, in addition to sitting meditation, yoga, and mindful walking, a good deal of mindful kayaking. The retreat took place on isolated outer islands in the vast Tebenkof Bay Wilderness Area in southeast Alaska, reached by float plane. When we got back to town after eight days in the wilderness, the cover story of *Time* magazine (August 4, 2003) was on meditation. The very fact that it was a cover story featuring detailed descriptions of the effects of meditation on the brain and on health was a bellwether of how meditation has entered and has been embraced by the mainstream of our culture. It is no longer a marginal engagement on the part of the very few or the easily dismissed as crazy. There was another *Time* cover story on mindfulness and MBSR in 2014. By then, it was being touted as "The Mindful Revolution."

Indeed, meditation centers are sprouting up everywhere, offering retreats and classes and workshops, and even stopping-in-on-the-way-to-work sittings, and more and more people are coming to them to learn and to practice together. Yoga has never been more popular,

---

* See Mumford, G. *The Mindful Athelete: Secrets to Pure Performance* (Parallel Press, Berkeley, CA), 2015.

and is passionately being taken up by children and by seniors and everybody in between. And now there are impressive online mindfulness summits, right at your fingertips, with many skilled and experienced presenters, as well as excellent podcasts that help whoever is interested to get more deeply into mindfulness from different perspectives, including neuroscience, medicine and health care, and psychology.

What on earth is going on?

You might say that we are in the early stages of waking up as a culture to the potential of deep intimacy with interiority, to the power of cultivating awareness and learning to inhabit stillness and silence. We are beginning to realize the power of the present moment to bring us greater clarity and insight, greater emotional stability, and wisdom, an embodied wisdom that we can carry into the world, into our families and our work, into society more broadly, and into the domain of the global. In a word, meditation is no longer something foreign and exotic to our culture. It is now as American as anything else. Or English, or French, or Italian, or South American. It has arrived. And none too soon either, given the state of the world and the huge forces impinging on our lives. It may just be (and I like to think it is) the beginning of a Renaissance of wakefulness, compassion, and wisdom expressing itself globally through an infinite number of different forms.

But again, please keep one thing in mind…It's not what you think!

Original Moments

There was a time from the early to late seventies when I studied with a Korean Zen Master named Seung Sahn. His name translates literally as High Mountain, the name of the mountain in China where the sixth Zen Patriarch, Hui Neng, is said to have attained enlightenment. We called him Soen Sa Nim, which I only much later found out means honored Zen teacher. I don't think any of us actually knew what it meant at the time. It was just his name.

He had come over from Korea and somehow wound up in Providence, Rhode Island, where some Brown University students "discovered" him, improbably (but we came to learn pretty much everything with him was improbable) repairing washing machines in a small shop owned by some fellow Koreans. These students organized an informal group around him to find out what this guy was all about and had to offer. Those small informal gatherings eventually gave birth to the Providence Zen Center and from there, in the decades that followed, to many other centers around the world that supported Soen Sa Nim's teachings. I heard about him from a student of mine at Brandeis, and went down to Providence one day to check him out.

There was something about Soen Sa Nim that was utterly fascinating. First, he was a Zen Master, whatever that was, who was repairing washing machines and seemingly very happy doing so. He had a perfectly round face that was disarmingly open and winsome. He was utterly present, utterly himself, no airs, no conceit. His head was completely shaved (he called hair "ignorance grass" and said for monks it had to be cut regularly). He wore funny thin white rubber slip-on shoes that looked like little boats (Korean monks don't wear leather because it comes from animals), and in the early days mostly hung out in his underwear, although when he taught, he wore long gray robes and a simple brown kesha, a flat square of material sewn from many pieces of cloth that hung around his neck and rested on his chest, symbolical in Zen of the tattered robes of the first Zen practitioners in China. He also had fancier and more colorful outfits for special occasions and ceremonies, which he performed for the local Korean Buddhist community.

He had an unusual way of speaking, in part because he didn't know many words in English at first, and in part because American grammar eluded him completely. And so he spoke in a kind of broken English Korean that got his points across in just unbelievable ways that entered the mind of the listener with a breathtaking freshness because our minds had never heard thinking like that and so couldn't process it in the ordinary ways we usually do with what is heard. As tends to happen in such circumstances, many of his students fell into talking among themselves in the same way, in broken English, saying things to each other like "Just go straight, don't check your mind," and "The arrow is already downtown," and "Put it down, just put it down," and "You already understand," things like that that made sense to them but sounded insane to anyone else.

Soen Sa Nim was maybe five feet ten inches tall, not thin but not rotund either. Perhaps corpulent describes him best. He seemed ageless but was probably in his mid-forties. He was well known and highly respected in Korea, it was said, but had apparently chosen to come to America and bring his teachings to where the action was in those days. American youth in the early seventies certainly had a lot of energy and enthusiasm for Eastern meditative traditions, and he was part of a large wave of Asian meditation teachers who came to America in the sixties and seventies. If you want to get a flavor for his verbatim teachings in those days, you can read *Dropping Ashes on the Buddha*, by Stephen Mitchell.

Soen Sa Nim would often begin a public talk by taking the "Zen" stick he usually had within reach, fashioned from a gnarled and twisted, highly polished burl of demented tree branch, which he sometimes leaned his chin on as he peered out at the audience and, holding it up in the air horizontally above his head, bellow: "Do you see this?" Long silence. Puzzled looks. Then he would bang it straight down on the floor or on a table in front of him. It would make a loud thwack. "Do you hear this?" Long silence. More puzzled looks.

Then he would begin his talk. Often he didn't explain what that opening gambit was all about. But the message slowly became clear, maybe only after seeing him do this time and time again. No need to make things complicated where Zen or meditation or mindfulness are concerned. Meditation is not aimed at developing a fine philosophy of life or mind. It is not about thinking at all. It is about keeping things simple. Right now, in this moment, do you see? Do you hear? This seeing, this hearing, when unadorned, is the recovery of original mind, free from all concepts, including "original mind." And it is already here. It is already ours. Indeed, it is impossible to lose.

If you do see the stick, who is seeing? If you do hear the hit, who is hearing? In the initial moment of seeing, there is just the seeing, before thinking sets in and the mind secretes thoughts like: "I wonder what he means?" "Of course I see the stick." "That is quite a stick." "I don't think I ever saw a stick like that." "I wonder where he got it." "Maybe Korea." "It would be nice to have a stick like that." "I get what he is doing with that stick." "I wonder if anybody else does?" "This is kind of cool." "Wow!" "Meditation is pretty far out." "I could really get with this." "I wonder what I would look like in those robes."

Or with the hearing of the loud bang: "This is a peculiar way to start a talk." "Of course, I heard the sound." "Does he think we are deaf?" "Did he actually hit that table?" "He must have left quite a mark in it." "That was some wallop." "How could he do that?" "Doesn't he know that that is somebody's property?" "Doesn't he care?" "What kind of a person is he anyway?"

That was the whole point.

"Do you see?" We hardly ever just see.

"Do you hear?" We hardly ever just hear.

Thoughts, interpretations, and emotions pour in so quickly following any and every experience—and as expectations even before the experience arises—that we can hardly say that we were "there" at all for the original moment of seeing, the original moment of hearing. If we were, it would be "here," and not "there."

Instead, we see our concepts rather than the stick. We hear our concepts, rather than the thwack. We evaluate, we judge, we digress, we categorize, we react emotionally, and so quickly that the moment of pure seeing, the moment of pure hearing, is lost. For that moment at least, you could say that we have lost our minds and have taken leave of our senses.

Of course, such moments of unawareness color what comes next, so there is a tendency to stay lost, to fall into automatic patterns of thinking and feeling for long stretches of time and not even know it.

So, when Soen Sa Nim asked "Do you see this? Do you hear this?" it was not as trivial as it might have appeared to be at first blush. He was inviting us to wake up from the dream of our self-absorption and our endless spinning out of stories that distance us from what is actually happening in these moments that add up to what we call our life.

Odysseus and the Blind Seer

We sometimes say "Come to your senses!" to enjoin somebody to wake up to how things actually are. Usually though—you may have noticed—people don't magically get sensible just because we are imploring them to. (Nor do we when we implore ourselves.) Their whole orientation—to themselves, the situation, and everything else—may need an overhaul, sometimes a drastic one. How to go about that? Sometimes it takes a health crisis to wake us up—if it doesn't kill us first.

We say "He has taken leave of his senses" to mean he is no longer in touch with reality. Most of the time, it is not so easy to get back in touch. Where would one even start when you are already so off? And what if the whole society or the whole world has taken leave of its senses, so that everybody is focusing on some aspect of the elephant but nobody is apprehending the whole of it? Meanwhile, what we thought was an elephant is morphing into something more like a monster running amok, and we are stuck unwilling to perceive and name what is so, much like the spectator-citizens in the realm of the duped emperor with his new set of invisible "clothes."

The fact of the matter is that it is not so easy to come to our senses without practice. And as a rule, we are colossally out of practice. We are out of shape when it comes to our senses. We are out of shape when it comes to recognizing our relationship with those aspects of body and mind that partake of the senses, are co-extensive with the senses, are informed by the senses, and are shaped by them. In other words, we are colossally out of shape when it comes to perception and awareness, whether oriented outwardly or inwardly or both. We get back in shape by exercising our faculties for paying attention over and over again, just like a muscle. And what grows stronger and more robust and flexible through such workouts, often in the face of considerable resistance from within our own mind, is a lot more interesting than, say, a bicep.

Most of the time, our senses, including of course our minds, are playing tricks on us, just from force of habit and the fact that the senses are not passive but require coherent active assessment and interpretation from various regions of the brain. We see, but we are scantly aware of seeing as *relationship*, the relationship between our capacity to see and what is available to be seen. We believe what we think is in front of us. But that experience is actually filtered through our various unconscious thought constructs and the mysterious way that we seem to be alive inside a world that we can take in through the eyes.

So we see some things, but at the same time, we may not see what is most important or most relevant for our unfolding life. We see habitually, which means we see in very limited ways, or we don't see at all, even sometimes what is right under our noses and in front of our very eyes. We see on automatic pilot, taking the miracle of seeing for granted, until it is merely part of the unacknowledged background within which we go about our business.

We can have children and go for years without really seeing them because we are only "seeing" our thoughts about them, colored by our expectations or our fears. The same can be true for any or all of our relationships. We live within the natural world, but much of the time we don't notice it either, missing the way sunlight might be reflecting off of one particular leaf, or how surrounded we are in the city by amazingly misshapen reflections in windows and windshields. Nor do we sense, as a rule, that we are being seen and sensed by others, including wildlife in the landscape—you'd know it better spending the night in a rain forest—and in ways that might very much diverge from our own view of ourselves.

Perhaps such pervasive and endemic blindness on our part as human beings is one reason Homer, at the very dawn of the Western literary tradition, crafting his orally transmitted tale circa 800 BCE, in the middle of *The Odyssey*, has Odysseus seek out Tiresias on the border of Hades to learn his fate and what he must do to return safely home. For Tiresias is a blind seer and whenever a "blind seer" makes an appearance, you know things are about to get more interesting and more real. Homer seems to be telling us that real seeing goes way beyond having functional eyes. In fact, functioning eyes can be an impediment to finding one's way. We must learn how to see beyond our own habitual and characterological blindnesses, in Odysseus's case the product of his arrogance and wiliness, which were both his strength and his undoing, and therefore, an incomparable gift to reckon with and learn from.*

Not only do we not see what is here, often we see what is not here. How the eye fabricates! The mind makes things up. In part, this is due to our wildly creative imagination. In part, it's the way our

---

* Indeed, Tiresias predicts a second voyage of Odysseus at the end of his life, this one a journey he will make alone, without his band of warriors, a solitary journey into the interior, carrying an oar on his shoulder, until he is finally asked by a stranger who has never seen the sea, "What is that winnowing fan on your shoulder?" A winnowing fan was used in the ancient world to separate wheat from chaff, a symbol here of wise discernment, of a wisdom Odysseus will only come to long after his odyssey is at an end, his wife's suitors destroyed, his realm restored. This inward journey of his later years is forecast by the blind seer and is never mentioned by Homer again. According to Helen Luke, who dared to write the story Homer never told, it presages the journey of old age, toward wisdom and inner peace, and a reconciliation with the gods, who are offended by our own blindness and hubris.

nervous system is wired up. Is there a triangle in the figure below, known as the Kanizsa triangle, or not? Soen Sa Nim would say: "If you say there is, I will hit you [with his Zen stick] thirty times [he didn't really, but in the old days in China, they did]. If you say there isn't, I will hit you thirty times. What can you do?" He didn't use Kanizsa triangles, but any object that was handy. "If you say this is/isn't a stick, a glass, a watch, a rock, I will hit you....What can you do?" It sure taught us not to be attached to form or emptiness, or at least, not to show it. But in spite of ourselves, show it we did much of the time, and just blundered through, hoping somehow to learn and grow in the process, from the caring that went into his apparent lack of caring, if from nothing else.

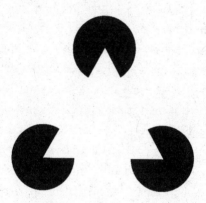

We all know that when it comes to perceiving through our eyes, we see certain things but not others, even when they are staring us right in the face. And we can be easily conditioned to see in certain ways and prevented from seeing in others. Slight-of-hand magicians make use of this selectivity in our observing all the time. Their art just baffles—and delights—the mind by skillfully diverting our attention and wreaking havoc with the senses.

More universally, people in different cultures can see the same event very differently, depending on their belief systems and orientation. They are seeing through different mind lenses and therefore seeing different realities. None are entirely true. Most are only true to a degree. Were Americans the liberators of Iraq or its oppressors? Be careful what you say. How attached are we to one view only, one that may be only partially true, only true to a degree?

We are all wont at times to fall mindlessly into black-and-white thinking, going for the absolutes. It makes us feel better, more secure, but it is also hugely blinding. This is good. That is bad. This is right. That is wrong. We are strong. They are weak. We are smart, they are not. She's a peach. He's a pain. I'm a wreck. They are nuts. He'll never grow out of it. She's so insensitive. I'll never be able to do this. It's unstoppable.

All of these statements are thoughts, and they tend to be view-distorting and limiting, even if they are partly true. Because for the most part, things in the real world are only true to a degree. There is no such thing as a tall person. One is only tall to a degree. No such thing as a smart person. One is only smart to a degree. But when we fall into such thinking, if we examine it in the light of a larger awareness, we find it tends to be rigid, confining, and inevitably, at least partly wrong. Thus, our black-and-white, either/or seeing and thinking leads rapidly to fixed and limiting judgments, often arrived at reflexively, automatically, without reflection, often thwarting our ability to steer our way "home" through the vagaries of life. *Discernment,* on the other hand, as differentiated from *judging,* leads us to see, hear, feel, perceive infinite shades of nuance, shades of gray between all-white and all-black, all-good or all-bad, and this what we might call "wise discerning" allows us to see and navigate through different openings whereas our quick-reaction judgments put us at risk for not seeing such openings at all, and missing the full spectrum of the real, and thus lead us to automatically and unwittingly limit the possible.

There is a whole field of mathematics and engineering based

on this complex fractal patterning in the world in-between all one way and all another way. It is called fuzzy math. The funny thing is, the more you start paying attention to the degreeness of things, the clearer the mind gets, not the fuzzier. It will be helpful as we move more and more deeply into the exploration of mindfulness to keep this in mind. Bart Kosko of the University of Southern California, in his book *Fuzzy Thinking*, points out that the world of zero and one, black and white, is the world as articulated by Aristotle, who, parenthetically, also described the five senses in writing for the first time in Western culture. All the shades of gray, as well as zero and one, are the world as articulated by the Buddha. So which model of the world is correct?

Be careful!

Apples can be red, green, or yellow. But if you look closely, they are only red, or green, or yellow to a degree. Sometimes there are bigger or smaller splotches or specks of the other colors mixed in. No natural apple is entirely red, or green, or yellow. The meditation teacher Joseph Goldstein recounts the story of the elementary school teacher who asked her class, "What color is this, children?" as she held up an apple. Many children said red, some said yellow, some said green, but one boy said, "White." "White?" said the teacher. "Why are you saying white? You can plainly see it is not white." At which point the boy comes up to the desk, takes a bite out of it, and holds it up for the teacher and the class to see.

Goldstein is also fond of pointing out that there is no Big Dipper in the sky, just the appearance of a big dipper from our particular angle on those stars. But it sure looks like a big dipper when you look up on a dark night. And this non–big dipper still helps us to locate the North Star and navigate by it.

Before reading further, pause and explore the drawing on the next page. What do you see?

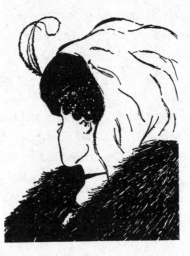

Some people see an old woman and only an old woman. Others see a young woman and only a young woman. Which is it? If, prior to showing the above drawing, I flash the picture on the left of page 34 for even five seconds to half of a large audience while the other half have their eyes closed, those people are much more likely to see a young woman in the above drawing than the other half, who were flashed the picture on the right of page 34. They, in contrast, are much more likely to see an old woman in the above drawing. Once the pattern is set, it is very hard for some people to see the other one, even after staring at it for a long time, unless they are shown both of these unambiguous sketches.

And then there is the enchanting story from Antoine de St.-Exupéry's marvelous fantasy, *Le Petit Prince*:

> Once when I was six I saw a magnificent picture in a book about the jungle, called *True Stories*. It showed a boa constrictor swallowing a wild beast...
>
> In the book, it said: "Boa constrictors swallow their prey whole, without chewing. Afterward they are no longer able to move, and they sleep during the six months of their digestion."

In those days I thought a lot about jungle adventures, and eventually managed to make my first drawing, using a colored pencil. My drawing Number One looked like this:

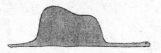

I showed the grown-ups my masterpiece and I asked them if my drawing scared them.

They answered: "Why be scared of a hat?"

My drawing was not a picture of a hat. It was a picture of a boa constrictor digesting an elephant. Then I drew the inside of the boa constrictor, so the grown-ups could understand. They always needed explanations. My drawing Number Two looked like this:

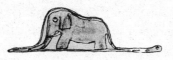

The grown-ups advised me to put away my drawings of boa constrictors, outside or inside, and apply myself instead to geography, history, arithmetic, and grammar. That is why I abandoned, at the age of six, a magnificent career as an artist. I had been discouraged by the failure of my drawing Number One and of my drawing Number Two. Grown-ups never understand anything by themselves, and it is exhausting for children to have to provide explanations over and over again.

So to come to our senses, perhaps we will need to develop and learn to trust our innate capacity to see beneath the surface of appearances to more fundamental dimensions of reality, as Tiresias, who was blind yet could see what was important, was embodying for Odysseus, who

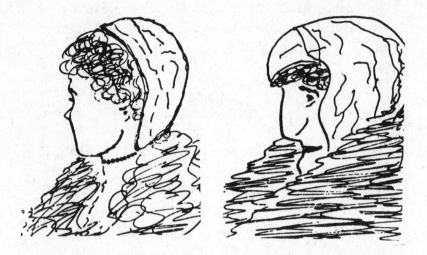

was not literally blind but couldn't discern what he most needed to see and know. Perhaps these new dimensions that only seem hidden from us can help us wake up to the full spectrum of our experience of the world, and our potential to understand ourselves and find ways to be and to be of use that nourish both ourselves and the world, and that call forth from us what is deepest and best in ourselves, and most human.

*

My inside, listen to me, the greatest spirit,
the teacher, is near,
wake up, wake up!

Run to his feet—
he is standing close to your head right now.
You have slept for millions and millions of years.
Why not wake up this morning?

KABIR
Translated by Robert Bly

No Attachments

There is a joke making the rounds that goes like this:

Have you heard the one about the Buddhist vacuum cleaner?
    Are you kidding? What on earth is a Buddhist vacuum cleaner?
    You know! No attachments!

The fact that people get this at all suggests that the core message of Buddhist meditation has found its way into the collective psyche of our culture. From the perspective of the era of my childhood in the 1940s and '50s, this cultural mind enlargement would have been highly improbable, even inconceivable. Carl Jung remarked as much in commenting about the potential difficulty for the Western mind to understand Zen, even though he himself had the highest respect for its aims and methods.

Nevertheless, the shift has already occurred, and maybe Jung's abiding interest in it in an earlier era was emblematical of what is unfolding now, as well as instrumental. Still, he would have been astonished by how deeply mindfulness and dharma wisdom have penetrated the mainstream world.

The historian Arnold Toynbee is said to have commented that the coming of Buddhism to the West would be seen in time as the single most important historical event of the twentieth century. That is a staggering assertion given all the remarkable events of that one hundred years, including all the untold suffering that humans inflicted upon each other. Whether he was correct or not remains to be seen. It will probably require the perspective of at least another hundred years or so to even venture an informed assessment. But something is clearly happening on this front.

In any event, nowadays people get the vacuum cleaner joke, and many others that find their way into the *New Yorker* and such places in the form of cartoons about meditation. Here's one:

> Two monks in robes who have obviously just finished a period of sitting meditation. One turns toward the other. The caption reads: "Are you not thinking what I'm not thinking?"

The culture is catching a certain drift about meditation. And it is hardly limited to high-brow culture. We find it in bubble gum comics, movies, and advertisements on subway walls, magazines, and newspapers. Inner peace is now used to sell just about everything, from spa vacations to new cars to perfume to bank accounts. No one is saying this is a good thing, but it does indicate that something is shifting as we become more aware on some level of the promise and the practical reality of such pursuits, and of course, of our capacity to exploit just about anything for the sake of marketing a product.

In one bubble gum comic given to me years ago by a young patient, the sequence of pictures is accompanied by the following dialogue. From the text, you can imagine for yourself what the pictures might be:

> "What are you up to, Mort?"
> "I'm practicing meditation. After a few minutes, my mind is a complete blank."
> "Gee, and I thought he was born that way."

That meditation is about making the mind go blank is a complete misunderstanding of meditation. Even so, whatever people construe it to be, meditation is out there in Western culture as never before. For years, the Dalai Lama's face peered down from huge billboards, courtesy of Apple Computer. I go into my local Staples to buy office supplies and there is his book *The Art of Happiness* in its own display, in the business section no less. Something profound has happened over the past forty years, and the seeds of it are now sprouting all over the place. It could be called the coming of Dharma to the West. If the word "dharma" is unfamiliar to you, or its meaning opaque at the moment, we will be exploring it in some detail in Part 2. For now, suffice it to say that it can be thought of as both the formal teachings of the Buddha (with a capital D) and also a universal, ethical, intrinsic lawfulness describing the way things are and the nature of the mind that perceives and knows (with a small d).

The Buddha once said that the core message of all his teachings—he taught continually for over forty-five years—could be summed up in one sentence. On the off chance that that might be the case, it might not be a bad idea to commit that sentence to memory. You never know when it might come in handy, when it might make sense to you even though in the moment before, it really didn't. That sentence is:

"Nothing is to be clung to as I, me, or mine."

In other words, no attachments. Especially to fixed ideas of yourself and who you are.

It is a hard message to swallow at first blush because it brings into question everything that we think we are, which for the most part seems to come from what we identify with, our bodies, our thoughts, our feelings, our relationships, our values, our work, our expectations of what is "supposed" to happen and how things are "supposed" to work out for me in order for me to be happy, our stories of where we came from and where we are going and of who we are.

But let's not react quite so quickly, even though at first blush the Buddha's counsel may feel more than a little scary or even stupid or irrelevant. For the operative word here is "clinging." It is important to understand what is meant by clinging so we don't misinterpret this injunction as a disavowal of all we hold dear, when in fact it is an invitation to come into greater touch and into a direct, living contact with everybody we hold dear to our hearts and everything that is most important to our well-being as a whole person, body, mind, soul, and spirit, whatever language you want to use. That includes what is difficult to handle or come to terms with—the stress and anguish of the human condition itself when it rears up in our lives, as it is apt to do sooner or later, in one way or another. It is saying that it is our attachment to the thoughts we have of who we are that may be the impediment to living life fully, and a stubborn obstacle to any realization of who and what we actually are, and of what is important, and possible. It may be that in clinging to our self-referential ways of seeing and being, to the parts of speech we call the personal pronouns, "I," "me," and "mine," we sustain the unexamined habit of grasping and clinging to what is not fundamental, all the while missing or forgetting what is.

The Origin of Shoes: A Tale

There is an ancient story of how shoes came to be invented.

Once upon a time, a long long time ago, it seems, there was a princess who, while walking one day, stubbed her toe on a root sticking out in the path. Vexed, she went to the prime minister and insisted that he draw up an edict declaring that the entire kingdom should be paved in leather so that no one would ever have to suffer from stubbing a toe again. Now the prime minister knew that the king always wanted to please his daughter in any and every way, and so might be appealed to to actually cover the kingdom in leather, which, while it might solve that problem and make the princess happy and save everybody from the indignity of stubbed toes, would be sorely problematic in many ways, to say nothing of expensive. Thinking quickly [I won't say "on his feet"], the prime minister responded: "I have it! Instead of covering the whole kingdom in leather, Your Highness, why don't we craft pieces of leather shaped to your feet and attach them in some suitable way? Then, wherever you go, your feet will have protection at the point of contact with the ground, and we will not have to incur such a large expense and forgo the sweetness of the earth." The princess was well pleased with this suggestion, and so shoes came into the world, and much folly was averted.

I find this story quite enchanting. It reveals several profound insights about our minds in the guise of a simple children's tale. First, things happen to us that generate vexations and aversion, two words Buddhists in some traditions love to use and which I think, in spite of their quaint ring, really do accurately describe our emotions when things don't go "our way." We stub our toe and we don't like it. Right then and there, we do get vexed, feel thwarted, and fall into aversion. We might even say, "I hate stubbing my toe." Right then and there, we make it into a something, a problem, usually "my" problem, and then the problem needs a solution. If we are not careful, the solution can be far worse than the problem. Second, wisdom is suggesting that the place to apply the remedy is at the point of contact, in the very moment of contact. We guard against stubbed toes by wearing protection on our feet, not by covering over the whole world out of our ignorance, desire, fear, or anger.

Similarly, we can guard against the elaborate cascade of often vexing or enthralling thoughts and emotions commonly triggered by even one bare sense impression. We can do so by bringing our attention to the point of contact, in the moment of contact with the sense impression. In this way, when there is seeing, the eyes are momentarily in contact with the bare actuality of what is seen. In the next moment, all sorts of thoughts and feelings pour in…"I know what that is." "Isn't it lovely." "I don't like it as much as I liked that other one." "I wish it would stay this way." "I wish it would go away." "Why is it here to annoy, thwart, frustrate me in this moment?" And on and on and on.

The object or situation is just what it is. Can we see it with open bare attention in the very moment of seeing, and then bring our awareness to see the triggering of the cascade of thoughts and feelings, liking and disliking, judging, wishing, remembering, hoping, fearing and panicking that follow from the original contact like night follows day?

If we are able, even for one moment, to simply rest in the seeing of what is here to be seen, and vigilantly apply mindfulness right in the moment of contact, we can become alerted to the cascade of thoughts and reactions as it begins, unleashed by the experience of its being either pleasant, unpleasant, or neutral—and choose not to be caught up in it, whatever its characteristics. Instead, we can allow it to just unfold as it is, without pursuit if it is pleasant or rejection if it is unpleasant. In that very moment, the vexations actually can be seen to dissolve because they are simply recognized as mental phenomena arising in the mind. Applying mindfulness in the moment of contact, at the point of contact, we can rest in the openness of pure seeing, without getting so caught up in our highly conditioned, reactive, and habitual thinking or in a stream of disturbance in the feeling realm, which of course only leads to more disturbance and turbulence of mind, and carries us away from any chance of appreciating the bare actuality of what is, or, for that matter, of responding to it in an effective and authentic way.

Mindfulness thus serves as our shoes, protecting us from the consequences of our own habits of emotional reaction, forgetfulness, and unconscious harming that stem from not recognizing, remembering, and inhabiting the deeper nature of our own being in the moment in which a sense impression, any sense impression, arises.

With mindfulness applied in that moment and in that way, at the point of contact, in the arising itself, the nature of our seeing, the miracle of our seeing, is free to be what it is, and the mind's essential nature is not disturbed. For that moment, we are free from harm, free from all conceptualizing, and from all vestiges of clinging. We are merely resting in the knowing of what is seen, heard, smelled, tasted, felt, or thought—whether pleasant, unpleasant, or neutral. Stringing moments of mindfulness together in this way allows us to gradually rest more and more in a non-conceptual, a more non-reactive, a more choiceless awareness, to actually *be* the knowing that awareness already is, to *be* its spaciousness, its freedom.

Not bad for a pair of cheap shoes.

Actually, they are not so cheap. They are priceless; also invaluable. They cannot even be bought, only crafted out of our pain and our wisdom. They wind up, in T. S. Eliot's words, "costing not less than everything."

MEDITATION—IT'S NOT WHAT YOU THINK

It might be good to clarify a few common misunderstandings about meditation right off the bat. First, meditation is best thought of as a way of being rather than a technique or a collection of techniques.

I'll say it again.

Meditation is a way of being, not a technique.

This doesn't mean that there aren't methods and techniques associated with meditation practice. There are. In fact, there are hundreds of them, and we will be making good use of some of them. But without understanding that all techniques are orienting vehicles pointing at ways of being, ways of being in relationship to the present moment and to one's own mind and one's own experience, we can easily get lost in techniques and in our misguided but entirely understandable attempts to use them to get somewhere else and experience some special result or state that we think is the goal of it all. As we shall see, such an orientation can seriously impede our understanding of the full richness of meditation practice and what it offers us. So it is helpful to just keep in mind that above all, meditation is a way of being, or, you could say, a way of seeing, a way of knowing, even a way of loving.

Second, meditation is not relaxation spelled differently. Perhaps I should say that again as well: Meditation is not relaxation spelled differently.

That doesn't mean that meditation is not frequently accompanied by profound relaxation and by deep feelings of well-being. Of course it is, or can be, sometimes. But mindfulness meditation is the embrace of any and all mind states in awareness, without preferring one to another. From the point of view of mindfulness practice, pain or anguish, or for that matter boredom or impatience or frustration or anxiety or tension in the body are all equally valid objects of our attention if we find them arising in the present moment, each a rich opportunity for insight and learning, and potentially, for liberation, rather than signs that our meditation practice is not "succeeding" because we are not feeling relaxed or experiencing calmness or bliss in some moment.

We might say that meditation is really a way of being appropriately in tune with the circumstances one finds oneself in, in any and every moment. If we are caught up in the preoccupations of our own mind, in that moment we cannot be present in an appropriate way or perhaps at all. We will bring an agenda of some kind to whatever we say or do or think, even if we don't know it.

This doesn't mean that there won't be various things going on in our minds, many of them chaotic, turbulent, painful, and confusing if we start training to become more mindful. It is only natural that there will be. That is the nature of the mind and of our lives at times. But we do not have to be caught by those things, or so caught up in them that they color our capacity to perceive the full extent of what is going on and what is called for (or color our capacity to perceive that we have no idea what is really going on or what might be called for). It is the non-clinging, and therefore the clear perceiving, and the willingness to act appropriately within whatever circumstances are arising that constitute this way of being that we are calling meditation.

It is not uncommon for people who know little of meditation except what they have gleaned from the media to harbor the notion that meditation is basically a willful inward manipulation, akin to throwing a switch in your brain, that results in your mind going completely blank. No more thought, no more worry. You are catapulted into *the* "meditative" state, which is always one of deep relaxation, peace, calm, and insight, often associated with concepts of "nirvana" in the public's mind.

This notion is a serious, if totally understandable, misperception. Meditation practice can be fraught with thought and worry and desire, and every other mental state and affliction known to frequent human beings. It is not the content of your experience that is important. What is important is our ability to be aware of that content, and even more, of the factors that drive its unfolding and the ways in which those factors either liberate us or imprison us moment by moment and year in, year out. So just to be clear about it, there is no one "mindful state" that we are aiming to achieve or attain. Any condition or state we find ourselves in in any moment, including anger or fear or sadness, can be held in awareness and thus be seen, met, known, and accepted as part of the actuality of that moment.

While there is no question that meditation can lead to deep relaxation, peace, calm, insight, wisdom, and compassion, and that the term "nirvana" actually refers to an important and verifiable dimension of human experience* and is not merely the name of an aftershave lotion or a fancy yacht, it is never what one thinks, and what one thinks is never the whole story. That is one of the mysteries and attractions of meditation. Yet sometimes even seasoned meditators forget that meditation is not about trying to get anywhere special, and can long for or strive for a certain result that will fulfill our desires and expectations. Even when we "know better," it can still come up at times, and we have to "re-mind" ourselves in those moments to let go of such concepts and desires, to treat them just like any other thoughts arising in the mind, to remember to cling to *nothing*, and maybe even

---

* The word actually means "extinguished," as with a fire that has completely burned itself out. When what we think of as ourself and our desires are completely extinguished, in other words, they no longer arise, that is nirvana.

to see that they are intrinsically empty, mere fabrications, however understandable, of what we might call the wanting mind.

Another common misconception is that meditation is a certain way of controlling one's thoughts, or having specific thoughts. While this notion, too, has a degree of truth to it, in that there are specific forms of discursive meditation that are aimed at cultivating specific qualities of being such as lovingkindness and equanimity, and positive emotions such as joy and compassion, our ways of thinking about meditation often make practicing more difficult than it needs to be and prevent us from coming to our experience of the present moment as it actually is rather than the way we might want it to be, and with an open heart and an open mind.

For meditation, and especially mindfulness meditation, is not the throwing of a switch and catapulting yourself anywhere, nor is it entertaining certain thoughts and getting rid of others. Nor is it making your mind blank or willing yourself to be peaceful or relaxed. It is really an inward gesture that inclines the heart and mind (seen as one seamless whole) toward a full-spectrum awareness of the present moment just as it is, accepting whatever is happening simply because it is already happening, and not taking any of it personally, or noticing how personally you are taking it and letting even that realization be held in awareness. This inner orientation is sometimes referred to in psychotherapy as "radical acceptance." Whatever we call it, adopting this relationship to experience is hard work, very hard work, especially when what is happening does not conform to our expectations, desires, and fantasies. And our expectations, desires, and fantasies are all-pervasive and seemingly endless. They can color everything, sometimes in very subtle ways that are not at all obvious, especially when they are about meditation practice and issues of "progress" and "attainment."

So meditation is not about trying to get anywhere else. It is about allowing yourself to be exactly where you are and as you are, and for the world to be exactly as it is in this moment as well. This is not so easy, since there is always something that we can rightly find fault with if we stay inside the echo-chamber of our thinking. And so there tends to be great resistance on the part of the mind and body to settle into things just as they are, even for a moment. That resistance to what is may be even more compounded if we are meditating because we hope that by doing so, we can effect change, make things different, improve our own lives, and contribute to improving the lot of the world.

That doesn't mean that your aspirations to effect positive change, make things different, improve your life and the lot of the world are inappropriate. Those are all very real possibilities. Just by meditating, by sitting down and being still, you *can* change yourself and the world. In fact, just by sitting down and being still, in a small but not insignificant way, you already have.

But the paradox is that you can only change yourself or the world if you get out of your own way for a moment, and give yourself over and trust in allowing things to be as they already are, without pursuing anything, especially goals that are products of your thinking. Einstein put it quite cogently: "The problems that exist in the world today cannot be solved by the level of thinking that created them." Implication: We need to develop and refine our mind and its capacities for seeing and knowing, for recognizing and transcending whatever motives and concepts and habits of unawareness may have generated or compounded the difficulties we find ourselves embroiled within, a mind that knows and sees in new ways, that is motivated differently. This is the same as saying we need to return to our original, untouched, unconditioned mind.

How can we do this? Precisely by taking a moment to get out of our own way, to get outside of the stream of thought and sit by the bank and rest for a while in things as they are underneath our thinking, or as Soen Sa Nim liked to say, "before thinking." That means being with what is for a moment and trusting what is deepest and best in yourself, even if it doesn't make any sense to your thinking mind. Since you are far more than the sum of your thoughts and ideas and opinions, including your thoughts of who you are and of the world and the stories and explanations you tell yourself about all that, dropping in on the bare experience of the present moment is actually dropping in on just the qualities you may be hoping to cultivate—because they all come out of awareness, and it is awareness that we fall into when we stop trying to get somewhere or to have a special feeling and instead allow ourselves to be where we are and with whatever we are feeling right now. Awareness itself is the teacher, the student, and the lesson.

So, from the point of view of awareness, any state of mind is a meditative state. Anger or sadness is just as interesting and useful and valid to look into as enthusiasm or delight, and far more valuable than a blank mind, a mind that is insensate, out of touch. Anger, fear, terror, sadness, resentment, impatience, enthusiasm, delight, confusion, disgust, contempt, envy, rage, lust, even dullness, doubt, and torpor, in fact all mind states and body states are occasions to know ourselves better if we can stop, look, and listen, in other words, if we can come to our senses and be intimate with what presents itself in awareness in any and every moment. The astonishing thing, so counterintuitive, is that nothing else needs to happen. We can give up trying to make something special occur. In letting go of wanting something special to occur, maybe we can realize that something very special is already occurring, and is always occurring, namely life emerging in each moment as awareness itself.

Two Ways to Think about Meditation

The Instrumental and the Non-instrumental

Having said that meditation is not a technique or set of techniques to achieve a particular state, but rather a way of being, it may be useful to realize that there are two apparently contradictory ways to think about meditation and what it is all about, and the mix is different for different teachers and in different traditions. You may find me purposefully using the language of both these ways simultaneously, because both are equally true and important, and the tension between them exceedingly creative and useful.

One approach is to think of meditation as instrumental, as a method, a discipline that allows us to cultivate, refine, and deepen our capacity to pay attention and to dwell in present-moment awareness. The more we practice the method, which could actually be a number of different methods, the more likely we are over time to develop greater stability in our ability to attend to any object or event that arises in the field of awareness, either inwardly or outwardly. This stability can be experienced in the body as well as in the mind, and is often accompanied by an increasing vividness of perception and a calmness in the observing itself. Out of such systematic practice, moments of clarity and insight into the nature of things, including ourselves, tend to arise naturally. In this way of looking at meditation, it *is* progressive; there is a vector to it that aims toward wisdom, compassion, and clarity, a trajectory that has a beginning, a middle, and an end, although the process can hardly be said to be linear, and sometimes feels like it consists of one step forward and six steps back. In this regard, it is not dissimilar to any other competency that we may develop by working at. And there are instructions and teachings to guide you all along the way.

This way of looking at meditation is necessary, important, and valid. But—and it is a big but—even though the Buddha himself worked hard at meditating for six years and broke through to an extraordinary realization of freedom, clarity, and understanding, this method-based way of describing the process is not in itself complete and can, by itself, give an erroneous impression of what meditation actually involves.

Just as physicists have been compelled by the results of their experiments and calculations to describe the nature of elementary particles in two complementary ways, one as particles, the other as waves, even though they are really one thing—but here language fails because at that level they are not really things but rather more like properties of energy and space at the core of all things at unthinkably minute levels—with meditation there is a second, equally valid, way to describe it, a description that is critical to a complete understanding of what meditation really is when we come to practice it.

This other way of describing meditation is that whatever "meditation" is, it is not instrumental at all. If it is a method, it is the method of no method. It is not a doing. There is no going anywhere, nothing to practice, no beginning, middle, or end, no attainment, and nothing to attain. Rather, it is the direct realization and embodiment in this very moment of who you already are, outside of time and space and concepts of any kind, a resting in the very nature of your being, in what is sometimes called the natural state, original mind, pure awareness, no mind, or simply emptiness. You are already everything you may hope to attain, so no effort of the will is necessary—even for the mind to come back to the breath—and no attainment is possible. You are already it. It is already here. Here is already everywhere, and now is already always. There is no time, no space, no body, and no mind, to paraphrase the

great Indian fifteenth century Sufi poet, Kabir. And there is no purpose to meditation—it is the one human activity (non-activity really)
that we engage in for its own sake—for no purpose other than to be
awake to what is actually so.

For example, how can you possibly "attain" your foot when it is
not apart from you in the first place? We would never even think to
attain our foot, because it is already here. The thinking mind makes
it into "a foot," a thing, but unless it is severed from the body, it is not
a separate entity with its own intrinsic existence. It is simply the end
of the leg, adapted for standing and walking upright. When we are
thinking, it is a foot, but when we are in awareness, outside, underneath, and beyond thinking, it is simply what it is. And you already
have it, or put differently, it is not other than you and never was. Same
for your eyes, ears, nose, tongue, and every other part of your body.
As St. Francis put it: "What you are looking for is who is looking."

By the same token, how can you possibly attain sentience, knowing, original mind, when original mind, to paraphrase Ken Wilber,
is reading these words? How can you come to your senses, when your
senses are already fully operative? Your ears *already* hear, your eyes
already see, your body *already* feels. It is only when we turn them
into concepts that we *de facto* sever them from the body of our being,
which by its very nature is undivided, already whole, already complete, already sentient, already awake.

These two ways of understanding what meditation is are complementary and paradoxical, just as are the wave and particle nature of
matter at the quantum level and below. That means that neither is
complete by itself. Alone, neither is completely true. Together, they
both become true.

For this reason, both descriptions are important to know of and
keep in mind from the very beginning of taking up the practice of
meditation, and especially mindfulness meditation. That way, we are
less likely to get caught on the horns of dualistic thinking, either striving too hard to attain what we already are, or claiming to already be

what we have not in actuality tasted and realized and have no way of drawing on, even though technically speaking it may be true and we are already it. It is not merely that we have the potential to become it, although relatively speaking, from the instrumental perspective, that is the case. We are it, but—we don't know it. It may be right under our noses, closer than close, but it remains hidden all the same.

These two descriptions inform each other. When we hold them both, even merely conceptually at first, then the effort we make at sitting, or in the body scan or the yoga, or in bringing mindfulness into all aspects of our lives, will be the right kind of effort, and we will have the right kind of attitude because we will remember that actually, in terms of the fundamental nature of life and mind, there is no place to go and no striving is necessary. In fact, striving can rapidly become counterproductive. Keeping this in mind, we will be more inclined to remember to be kind and gentle with ourselves, relaxed, accepting, and clear even in the face of turmoil in the mind or in the world. We will be less inclined to idealize our practice or get lost in "gaining fantasies" of where it will take us if we "do it right." We will be less entrained into the contortions of our own reactivity, more likely to let go into and be able to rest effortlessly in non-doing, in non-striving, in our original beginner's mind, in other words, in awareness itself, without an agenda other than to be awake to what is. This inhabiting of awareness with things exactly as they are is orthogonal to any kind of instructional set we may be, from the instrumental perspective, and rightly so, whispering in our own ear.

From the relative and temporal perspective, what the Buddha called "right [meaning wise] effort" is absolutely required, and we will learn that lesson and know it firsthand as we come to practice over days, weeks, months, years, and decades. For there is no question that we do get lost in the perpetual agitations of body and mind. There is no question that, when we sit down to meditate, we so often find that our attention span is short-lived and hard to sustain, and our awareness more often than not clouded over, the mind less than luminous and clear, objects of attention less than vivid, regardless of any self-talk about the mind's natural state and luminous empty nature. So it is crucial that we remind ourselves to stay seated rather than jump up as soon as the mind becomes bored or agitated; to come back to the breath, for instance, or to let go of a chain of thoughts that has carried us away; and to settle once again, and always, in awareness itself. For all of these, and ultimately whatever emerges in this present moment, become the real "curriculum" of the moment, the real "curriculum" of mindfulness, and of life itself.

After living with these two descriptions of meditation for a time, the instrumental and the non-instrumental, you will find that they slowly become comfortable old friends and allies. Practice gradually, or sometimes even suddenly, transcends all ideas of practice and effort, and whatever effort we put in is no longer effort at all, but really love. Our efforts become the embodiment of self-knowing, and thus, of wisdom. But it is also no big deal. We are it more than we do it, because there is no more substantial difference between us and awareness than there is between us and our foot. We are never without it.

And yet...the foot of a Mikhail Baryshnikov or a Martha Graham in their prime is not quite the same as that of us regular folk. Their feet "know" something ours may not, although in their very nature, they are the same. We can marvel at that sameness, and that difference. We can love it. And we can be it too. Because in essence, we already are.

Why Even Bother? The Importance of Motivation

If, from the meditative perspective, everything you are seeking is already here, even if it is difficult to wrap your thinking mind around that concept, if there really is no need to acquire anything or attain anything or improve yourself, if you are already whole and complete and by that same virtue so is the world, then why on earth bother meditating? Why would we want to cultivate mindfulness in the first place? And why use particular methods and practices, if they are all in the service of not getting anywhere anyway, and when, moreover, I've just finished saying that methods and practices are not the whole of it anyway?

The answer is that as long as the meaning of "everything you are seeking is already here" is only a concept, it is only a concept, just another nice thought. Being merely a thought, it is extremely limited in its capacity for transforming you, for manifesting the truth the statement is pointing to, and ultimately changing the way you carry yourself and act in the world.

More than anything else, I have come to see meditation as an act of love, an inward gesture of benevolence and kindness toward ourselves and toward others, a gesture of the heart that recognizes our perfection even in our obvious imperfection, with all our shortcomings, our wounds, our attachments, our vexations, and our persistent habits of unawareness. It is a very brave gesture: to take one's seat for a time and drop in on the present moment without adornment.

In stopping, looking, and listening, in giving ourselves over to all our senses, including mind, in any moment, we are in that moment embodying what we hold most sacred in life. Making the gesture, which might include assuming a specific posture for formal meditation, but could also involve simply becoming more mindful or more forgiving of ourselves, immediately re-minds us and re-bodies us. In a sense, you could say that it refreshes us, makes this moment fresh, timeless, freed up, wide open. In such moments, we transcend who we think we are. We go beyond our stories and all our incessant thinking, however deep and important it sometimes is, and reside in the seeing of what is here to be seen and the direct, non-conceptual knowing of what is here to be known, which we don't have to seek because it is already and always here. We rest in awareness, in the knowing itself which includes, of course, not knowing as well. We become the knowing and the not knowing, as we shall see over and over again. And since we are completely embedded in the warp and woof of the universe, there is really no boundary to this benevolent gesture of awareness, no separation from other beings, no limit to either heart or mind, no limit to our being or our awareness, to our openhearted presence. In words, it may sound like an idealization. Experienced, it is merely what it is, life expressing itself, sentience quivering within infinity, with things just as they are.

Resting in awareness in any moment involves giving ourselves over to all our senses, in touch with inner and outer landscapes as one seamless whole, and thus in touch with all of life unfolding in its fullness in any moment and in every place we might possibly find ourselves, inwardly or outwardly.

Thich Nhat Hanh, the Vietnamese Zen master, mindfulness teacher, poet, and peace activist, aptly points out that one reason we might want to *practice* mindfulness is that most of the time we are unwittingly practicing its opposite. Every time we get angry we get better at being angry and reinforce the anger habit. When it is really bad, we say we see red, which means we don't see accurately what is happening at all, and so, in that moment, you could say we have lost our mind. Every time we become self-absorbed, we get better at becoming self-absorbed and going unconscious. Every time we get anxious, we get better at being anxious. Practice does make perfect. Without awareness of anger or of self-absorption, or ennui, or any other mind state that can take us over when it arises, we reinforce those synaptic networks within the nervous system that underlie our conditioned behaviors and mindless habits, and from which it becomes increasingly difficult to disentangle ourselves, if we are even aware of what is happening at all. Every moment in which we are caught, by desire, by an emotion, by an unexamined impulse, idea, or opinion, in a very real way we are instantly imprisoned by the contraction within the habitual way we react, whether it is a habit of withdrawal and distancing ourselves, as in depression and sadness, or of erupting and getting emotionally "hijacked" by our feelings when we fall headlong into anxiety or anger. Such moments are always accompanied by a contraction in both the mind and the body.

But, and this is a huge "but," there is simultaneously a potential opening available here as well, a chance *not* to fall into the contraction—or to recover more quickly from it—*if* we can bring awareness to it. For we are locked up in the automaticity of our reaction and caught in its downstream consequences (i.e., what happens in the very next moment, in the world and in ourselves) only by our blindness in that moment. Dispel the blindness, and we see that the cage we thought we were caught in is already open.

Every time we are able to know a desire as desire, anger as anger, a habit as habit, an opinion as an opinion, a thought as a thought, a mind-spasm as a mind-spasm, or an intense sensation in the body as an intense sensation, we are correspondingly liberated. Nothing else has to happen. We don't even have to give up the desire or whatever it is. To see it and know it *as desire*, as whatever it is, is enough. In any given moment, we are either practicing mindfulness or, de facto, we are practicing mindlessness. When framed this way, we might want to take more responsibility for how we meet the world, inwardly and outwardly in any and every moment—especially given that there just aren't any "in-between moments" in our lives.

So meditation is both nothing at all—because there is no place to go and nothing to do—and simultaneously the hardest work in the world—because our mindlessness habit is so strongly developed and resistant to being seen and dismantled through our awareness. And it does require method and practice and effort to develop and refine our capacity for awareness so that it can tame the unruly qualities of the mind that make it at times so opaque and insensate.

These features of meditation, both as nothing at all and as the hardest work in the world, necessitate a high degree of motivation to practice being utterly present without attachment or identification. But who wants to do the hardest work in the world when you are already overwhelmed with more things to do than you can possibly get done—important things, necessary things, things you may be very attached to so you can build whatever it is that you may be trying to build, or get wherever it is that you are trying to get to, or even sometimes, just so you can get things over with and check them off your to-do list? And why meditate when it doesn't involve doing anyway, and when the result of all the non-doing is never to get anywhere but to be where you already are? What would I have to show for all my non-efforts, which nevertheless take so much time and energy and attention?

All I can say in response is that everybody I have ever met who has gotten into the practice of mindfulness and has found some way or other to sustain it in their lives for a period of time has expressed the feeling to me at one point or another, usually when things are at their absolute worst, that they couldn't imagine what they would have done without the practice. It is that simple really. And that deep. Once you practice, you know what they mean. If you don't practice, there is no way to know.

And of course, probably most people are first drawn to the practice of mindfulness because of their suffering, because of stress or pain of one kind or another and their dissatisfaction with elements of their lives that they somehow sense might be set right through the gentle ministrations of direct observation, inquiry, and self-compassion. Stress and pain thus become potentially valuable portals and motivators through which to enter the practice.

*

And one more thing. When I say that meditation is the hardest work in the world, that is not quite accurate, unless you understand that I don't just mean "work" in the usual sense, but also as play. Meditation is playful too. It is hilarious to watch the workings of our own mind, for one thing. And it is much too serious to take too seriously. Humor, playfulness, and undermining any hint of a pious attitude in yourself are critical elements of mindfulness practice. And besides, maybe it is *parenting* that is the hardest work in the world. But, if you are a parent, are mindfulness and parenting two different things?

I recently got a call from a physician colleague in his late forties who had undergone hip replacement surgery, surprising for his age, for which he needed an MRI before the operation took place. He recounted how useful the breath wound up being when he was swallowed by the machine. He said he couldn't even imagine what it would be like for a patient who didn't know about mindfulness and using the breath to stay grounded in such a difficult situation, although of course it happens every single day.

He also said that he was astonished by the degree of mindlessness that characterized many aspects of his hospital stay. He felt successively stripped of his status as a physician, and a rather prominent one at that, and then of his personhood and identity. He had been a recipient of "medical care," but on the whole, that care had hardly been caring. Caring requires empathy and mindfulness, and open-hearted presence, what I often call *heartfulness*,* often surprisingly lacking where one would think it would be most in evidence. After all, we do call it health *care*. It is staggering, shocking, and saddening that such stories are even now all too common, and that they come even from doctors themselves when they become patients and need care themselves.

Beyond the ubiquity of stress and pain operating in my own life, sometimes in the most rending of ways, as it is with all of us in various moments or life circumstances, my motivation to practice mindfulness is fairly simple: Each moment missed is a moment unlived. Each moment missed makes it more likely I will miss the next moment, and live through it cloaked in mindless habits of automaticity of thinking, feeling, and doing rather than living in, out of, and through awareness. I see it happen over and over again. Thinking in the service of awareness is heaven. Thinking in the absence of awareness can be hell. For mindlessness is not simply innocent or insensitive, quaint or clueless. Much of the time it is actively harmful, wittingly or unwittingly, both to oneself and to the others with whom we come in contact or share our lives. Besides, life is overwhelmingly interesting, revealing, and awe-provoking when we show up for it wholeheartedly and pay attention to the particulars, even in our most challenging or unwanted moments.

If we sum up all the missed moments, inattention can actually consume our whole life and color virtually everything we do and every choice we make or fail to make. Is this what we are living for, to miss and therefore misconstrue our very lives? I prefer going into the adventure every day with my eyes open, paying attention to what

---

* In most Asian languages, the word for *mind* and the word for *heart* are the same, so if you are not hearing or feeling "heartfulness" when you hear the word "mindfulness," you are not really understanding its full dimensionality and meaning.

is most important, even if I keep getting confronted at times with the feebleness of my efforts (when I think they are "mine") and the tenacity of my most deeply ingrained and robotic habits (when I think they are "mine"). I find it useful to meet each moment freshly, as a new beginning, to keep returning to an awareness of now over and over again, and let a gentle but firm perseverance stemming from the discipline of the practice keep me at least somewhat open to whatever is arising and behold it, apprehend it, accept it to whatever degree I can manage in that moment, look deeply into it, and learn whatever it might be possible to learn as the nature of the situation is revealed in the attending itself.

When you come right down to it, what else is there to do? If we are not grounded in our being, if we are not grounded in wakefulness, are we not actually missing out on the gift of our very lives and the opportunity to be of any real benefit to others?

It does help if I remind myself to ask my heart from time to time what is most important right now, in this moment, and listen very carefully for the response.

As Thoreau put it at the end of Walden, "Only that day dawns to which we are awake."

Aiming and Sustaining

A colleague coming off retreat said she thought meditation practice was all about aiming the attention and then sustaining that focus moment by moment. I wrote it off at the time as being pretty self-evident, almost trivial. Besides, it had too much of a sense of agency to it, I thought to myself, judgingly, too much of a sense of doing something, and therefore too much reliance on someone to be doing the doing. It took me years for the value of that insight to sink in and be revealed as fundamental.

For just as breathing doesn't necessitate a "someone" we have to think of as the "breather" in any fundamental way, although we can fabricate the thought of one (such as *"the breather—that must be me of course, I am breathing"*), aiming and sustaining don't necessitate someone to do the aiming or sustaining either, although again, we can artificially make one up, and are pretty much bound to do so at first out of our persistent habit of "selfing." But really, both aiming and sustaining come about naturally as we become more comfortable and practiced in resting in awareness itself, in what we might call "being the knowing."

Let's take the breath as an example. Breathing is fundamental to life. It is just happening. As a rule, we don't pay much attention to it unless we are choking or drowning, or have allergies or a bad cold. But imagine resting in an awareness of breathing. To do so requires first that we feel the breath and afford it a place in the field of awareness, which is always changing in terms of what the mind or the body or the world offers up to divert and distract our attention. We might be able to feel the breath, but in the next moment, it is forgotten in favor of something else. The aiming is here, but there is no sustaining. So we have to aim over and over again. Coming back, coming back, coming back to the breath over and over again. Every time noticing, noticing, noticing, noticing what is carrying our attention away.

The sustaining comes with the intention to allow sustaining. It requires considerable attentiveness to keep the focus on the breath sensations when our attention is so labile, so easily pulled elsewhere. Over days, weeks, months, and years, however, with wise and gentle attention to sustaining and a perseverance in our practice that comes out of our love for a greater authenticity which we sense is possible and perhaps vaguely missing in the conduct and unfolding of our very lives, we come to rest more easily in the breath, in the knowing of it from moment to moment as it is unfolding.

This sustaining is known in Sanskrit as *samadhi*, that focused quality of mind that is one-pointed, concentrated, and if not utterly unwavering, is at least relatively stable. Samadhi is developed and deepened as the normally agitated activity of our minds stills itself through the continued exercise of our ability to recognize when the mind has wandered off the agreed-upon object of attention, in this case the breath, and to bring it back over and over again, without judgment, reaction, or impatience. Simply aiming, sustaining, recognizing when the sustaining has evaporated, then re-aiming and again sustaining. Over and over and over and over again. Like the fins of a submarine or the keel on a sailboat, samadhi stabilizes and steadies the mind even in the face of its winds and waves, which gradually abate as they cease being fed by our inattention and our veritable addiction to their presence and content. With the mind relatively steady and unwavering, any object we hold in awareness becomes more vivid, is apprehended with greater clarity.

In the early stages, samadhi is more likely to reveal itself as a possible condition of our minds when we are part of a class or work-shop, even more so on an extended meditation retreat, when we intentionally sequester ourselves for a time from the usual hustle and bustle of life and its endless preoccupations, obligations, and occasions for distraction and face the actuality of what is on our mind when it is left alone, relatively speaking. Just to experience such sustained elemental stillness outwardly and the interior silence and relative calm that can accompany it is ample reason for arranging one's life to cultivate and bathe in this possibility from time to time. We may come to see that the waves and winds of the mind are not fundamental, just weather patterns we habitually get caught in and then lost in, thinking the content is what is most important, rather than the awareness within which the content of our minds can unfold.

Once you have tasted some degree of concentration and stability of focus in your attention, it is somewhat easier to settle into such stability of mind and reside within it at other times than on retreat, right in the midst of a busy life. Of course, this doesn't mean that everything in the mind will be calm and peaceful. We are visited over time by all sorts of mind states and body states, some pleasant, others unpleasant, others so neutral they may be hard to notice at all. But what is more calm and more stable is our ability to attend. It is the platform of our observing that becomes more stable. And with a degree of sustained calmness in our attending, if we don't cling to it for its own sake, invariably comes the development of insight, fueled and revealed by our awareness, by mindfulness itself, the mind's intrinsic capacity to know any and all objects of attention in any and every moment—as they are, beyond mere conceptual knowing through labeling and making meaning out of things through thinking.

Mindfulness discerns the breath as deep when it is deep. It discerns the breath as shallow when it is shallow. It knows the coming in and it knows the going out. It knows its impersonal nature in the same way that you know in some deep way that it is not "you" who is breathing—it is more that breathing is just happening. Mindfulness knows the impermanent nature of each breath. It knows any and all thoughts, feelings, perceptions, and impulses as they arise in and around and outside each and any breath. For mindfulness is the knowing quality of awareness, the core property of mind itself. It is strengthened by sustaining, and it is self-sustaining. Mindfulness is the field of knowing. When that field is stabilized by calmness and one-pointedness, the arising of the knowing itself is sustained, and the quality of the knowing strengthened.

That knowing of things as they are is called wisdom. It comes from trusting your original mind, which is nothing other than a stable, infinite, open awareness. It is a field of knowing that apprehends instantly when something appears or moves or disappears within its vastness. Like the field of the sun's radiance, it is always present, but it is often obscured by cloud cover, in this case, the self-generated cloudiness of the mind's habits of distraction, its endless proliferating of images, thoughts, stories, and feelings, many of them not quite accurate.

The more we practice aiming and sustaining our attention, the more we learn to rest effortlessly in the sustain, as when we depress the sustain pedal on a piano—the notes continue to reverberate long after the keys are struck.

The more we rest effortlessly in the sustain, the more the natural radiance of our very nature as simultaneously a localized and an infinite expression of wisdom and love reveals itself, no longer obscured from others or, more importantly, from ourselves.

PRESENCE

If you happen to stumble upon somebody who is meditating, you know instantly that you have come into the orbit of something unusual and remarkable. Because I lead meditation classes and retreats, I have that experience quite often. I look out sometimes at hundreds of people sitting in silence, on purpose, with nothing happening whatsoever except what is happening in the various interior landscapes of life unfolding in the moment for each and every person there. Someone passing by might think it strange to see a hundred people sitting in a room in silence, doing nothing—not for a brief moment but for minutes on end, maybe even for an hour at one time. At the same time, that person might very well be moved in some way by a palpable feeling of emanating presence that is an all-too-rare experience for any of us. If you were that person, even if you didn't have any idea of what was going on, you might easily find yourself inexplicably drawn to linger, to gaze upon such a gathering with great curiosity and interest, sharing in the energy field of the silence. It is intrinsically attractive and harmonizing. The feeling of an effortless alert attention behind such sitting in silence without moving is itself overpowering, as is the sense of intentionality embodied in such an assembly.

Attention and intention. Two hundred people present in mindful silence, unmoving, with no agenda other than to be present is a staggering manifestation of human goodness in its own right. It is deeply moving, this unmoving presence. But actually, I am moved by the very same feeling when I am in the presence of even one person sitting.

At any given time, in a room with several hundred meditators, some may be struggling and distracted, working at being present, which is different from being present, if only a hairbreadth away in any moment. Yet it can feel like an infinite gulf when one is thinking or striving or in pain. So inwardly there can be a lot of going back-and-forth, in and out of awareness, especially when the stability of one's attention is undeveloped and making for a rocky time of it. Usually this translates into outward restlessness, wiggling, shifting, and slumping.

But in those for whom a degree of concentration has developed, or who are naturally more concentrated and focused, a sense of presence actually emanates from them. A person can appear subtly illuminated from within. Sometimes the peacefulness of a face will move me to tears. Sometimes there is the slightest of smiles, hanging absolutely still in the passage of time, not the smile of "ha-ha," not that, not the smile of any subject, but precisely, in that moment, the absence of a subject. It is plain to see. No longer is the person just a person or a personality. He or she has become being, pure and simple. Just being. Just wakefulness. Just peace. And in being peace, in that moment the beauty of the person as pure being is unmistakable.

I don't need to actually see any of this to know it. I can feel it with my eyes closed. Sitting up front facing the retreatants, or on retreat myself, surrounded by other people all sitting in silence in a room for about an hour, I feel the presence and beauty of those in front of me or around me far more than if we were in conversation. Even though many may be in pain or struggling, their very willingness to be in the discomfort and open to it brings them into this field of presence, the field of mindfulness, of silent illumination.

When school teachers call attendance in classrooms around the world, the children, in whatever language, respond by saying the equivalent of "present," by which everybody agrees tacitly that, yes, the child is in the classroom, no mistake about it. The child thinks so, the parents think so, and the teacher thinks so. But much of the time, it is only the child's body that is in the classroom. The child's gaze may be out the window for long stretches, perhaps years at a time, seeing things that no one else is seeing. The child's psyche may be in the dreamland of fantasy or, if the child is fundamentally happy, only incarnating in the classroom occasionally, because she has more important karmic work to do. Or the child may be dwelling, unbeknownst to all, hidden in a nightmare of anxiety, plagued by demons of self-doubt or self-loathing or numbing turbulence the likes of which cannot be voiced in those kinds of settings, if ever, and which make presence and concentrating on tasks nigh impossible when the child's world is one of being consistently and regularly, or for that matter, episodically, abused, disregarded, or neglected.

Tibetans use the term "Kundun" when speaking of the Dalai Lama. Kundun means the Presence. It is neither a misnomer nor an exaggeration. In his presence, you become more present. I have had the occasion to observe him on multiple occasions over a period of days, in a room with a small number of people, often with complex scientific conversations and presentations going on, varying naturally in degrees of interest. But he appears to be right there all the time, not just in his thinking but in his feeling tone. He attends to the matter at hand, and I've noticed that all of us around him become not only more present, but more open and more loving, just by being in his presence. He interrupts when he doesn't understand. He ponders deeply, you can see it on his face. Closeted with scientists and senior monks and scholars, he regularly asks pointed questions during their presentations, to which a frequent response is: "Your Holiness, that is exactly the question we asked ourselves at this point, and the next experiment we decided to do." He may sometimes appear distracted, but usually I am fooled if I think so because he stays right on the point. But he does often look deep in thought, puzzled, or pondering a point. In the next moment, he can be very playful, radiating delight and kindness. You could say he was born this way, and that is a whole other story, of course, but these qualities are also the result of years of a certain kind of rigorous training of the mind and heart. He is the embodiment of that training, even though he would modestly say it is nothing, which is also more than passingly correct.

When asked why people respond to him so warmly, he once replied, "I have no special qualities. Perhaps it is because all my life I have meditated on love and compassion with all my strength of mind." Apparently he does that for four hours every morning, no matter what the demands of the coming day are or where he is, and again for a brief time at the end of the day. Imagine that.

To be present is far from trivial. It may be the hardest work in the world. And forget about the "may be." It *is* the hardest work in the world—at least to sustain presence. And the most important. When you do fall into presence—healthy children live in the landscape of presence much of the time—you know it instantly, feel at home instantly. And being home, you can let loose, let go, rest in your being, rest in awareness, in presence itself, in your own good company.

Kabir, the wild ecstatic poet of fifteenth-century India revered by Muslims and Hindus alike, has a ferocious way of framing the calling of presence, and how easily it can escape us:

*

Friend, hope for the Guest while you are alive.
Jump into experience while you are alive!
Think… and think… while you are alive.
What you call "salvation" belongs to the time before death.

If you don't break your ropes while you are alive,
do you think
ghosts will do it after?

The idea that the soul will join with the ecstatic
just because the body is rotten—
that is all fantasy.
What is found now is found then.
If you find nothing now,
you will simply end up with an apartment in the City of
 Death.
If you make love with the divine now, in the next life you will
 have the face of satisfied desire.

So plunge into the truth, find out who the Teacher is,
 Believe in the Great Sound!

Kabir says this: When the Guest is being searched for,
 it is the intensity of the longing for the Guest that
 does all the work.
Look at me, and you will see a slave of that intensity.

KABIR
translated by Robert Bly

A RADICAL ACT OF LOVE

In its outward manifestation, formal meditation appears to involve either stopping, by parking the body in a stillness that suspends activity, or giving oneself over to flowing movement. In either case, it is an embodiment of wise attention, an inward gesture undertaken for the most part in silence, a shift from doing to simply being. It is an act that may at first seem artificial but that we soon discover, if we keep at it, is ultimately one of pure love for the life unfolding within us and around us.

When I am guiding a meditation with a group of people, I often find myself encouraging them to throw out the thought "I am meditating" and just be awake, with no trying, no agenda, no ideas even about what it should look like or feel like or where your attention should be alighting...to simply be awake to what is in this very moment without adornment or commentary. Such wakefulness is not so easy to taste at first unless you are really in your beginner's mind,* but it is an essential dimension of meditation to know about from the very beginning, even if the experiencing of such open, spacious, choice-free awareness feels elusive in any particular moment.

---

* A phrase used by Suzuki Roshi, founder of the San Francisco Zen Center, to capture the innocence of an open and unencumbered inquiry on the meditation cushion into who you are and what the mind is via direct experience. "In the beginner's mind there are many possibilities, but in the expert's mind there are few."

Because we need to get simpler, not more complicated, it is hard for us at first to get out of our own way enough to taste this totally available sense of non-doing, of simply resting in being with no agenda, but fully awake. That is the reason that there are so many different methods and techniques for meditating, and so many different directions and instructions, what I sometimes refer to as "scaffolding." You might think of these methods as useful ways of intentionally and willfully bringing us back from a myriad of different directions and places in which we may be stuck, dazed, or confused, a bringing us back to utter and open silence, to what you might call our original wakefulness, which actually was never not here, is never not here, just as the sun is always shining and the ocean is always still at its depths.

> *I have a feeling that my boat*
> *has struck, down there in the depths,*
> *against a great thing.*
> > *And nothing*
> *happens! Nothing … Silence … Waves …*

> *—Nothing happens? Or has everything happened,*
> *and we are standing now, quietly, in the new life?*

JUAN RAMON JIMÉNEZ, "OCEANS"
Translated by Robert Bly

As the pace of our lives continues to accelerate, driven by a host of forces seemingly beyond our control, more and more of us are finding ourselves drawn to engage in meditation, in this radical act of being, this radical act of love, astonishing as that may seem given the materialistic "can do," speed-obsessed, progress-obsessed, celebrity-and-other-people's-lives-obsessed, social media-obsessed orientation of our culture. We are moving in the direction of meditative awareness for many reasons, not the least of which may be to maintain our individual and collective sanity, or recover our perspective and sense of meaning, or simply to deal with the outrageous stress and insecurity of this age. By stopping and intentionally falling awake to how things are in this moment, purposefully, without succumbing to our own reactions and judgments, and by working wisely with such occurrences with a healthy dose of self-compassion when we do succumb, and by our willingness to take up residency for a time in the present moment in spite of all our plans and activities aimed at getting somewhere else, completing a project or pursuing desired objects or goals, we discover that such an act is both immensely, discouragingly difficult and yet utterly simple, profound, hugely possible after all, and restorative of mind and body, soul and spirit right in that moment.

It is indeed a radical act of love just to sit down and be quiet for a time by yourself. Sitting down in this way is actually a way to take a stand in your life as it is right now, however it is. We take a stand here and now, by sitting down, and by sitting up.

It is the challenge of this era to stay sane in an increasingly insane world. How are we ever going to do it if we are continually caught up in the chatter of our own minds and the bewilderment of feeling lost or isolated or out of touch with what it all means and with who we really are when all the doing and accomplishing is sensed as being in some way empty, and we realize how short life is? Ultimately, it is only love that can give us insight into what is real and what is important. And so, a radical act of love makes sense—love for life and for the emergence of one's truest self.

Just to sit down and let ourselves drop into presence is a poignant and potent way of affirming that we are slowly but surely coming to our senses, and that that world of direct experience behind all the thinking and emotional reactions and all the self-absorption is still intact and utterly available to us for our succor, for our healing, and for our knowing how to be and, when we return to the doing, for knowing what to do and how to at least begin afresh.

Awareness and Freedom

Have you ever noticed that your awareness of pain is not in pain even when you are? I'm sure you have. It is a very common experience, especially in childhood, but one we usually don't examine or talk about because it is so fleeting and the pain so much more compelling in the moment it comes upon us.

Have you ever noticed that your awareness of fear is not afraid even when you are terrified? Or that your awareness of depression is not depressed; that your awareness of your bad habits is not a slave to those habits; or perhaps even that your awareness of who you are is not who you think you are?

You can test out any of these propositions for yourself any time you like simply by investigating awareness—by becoming aware of awareness itself. It is easy, but we hardly ever think to do it because awareness, like the present moment itself, is virtually a hidden dimension in our lives, embedded everywhere and therefore not so noticeable anywhere.

Awareness is immanent, and infinitely available, but it is camouflaged, like a shy animal. It usually requires some degree of effort and stillness if not stealth even to catch a glimpse of it, no less get a sustained look, even though it may be entirely out in the open. You have to be alert, curious, motivated to see it. With awareness, you have to be willing to let the knowing of it come to you, to invite it in, silently and skillfully in the midst of whatever you are thinking or experiencing. After all, you are already seeing; you are already hearing. There is awareness in all of that, coming through all the sense doors, including your mind, right here, right now.

If you move into pure awareness in the midst of pain, even for the tiniest moment, your relationship with your pain is going to shift right in that very moment. It is impossible for it not to change because the gesture of holding it, even if not sustained for long, even for a second or two, already reveals its larger dimensionality. And that shift in your relationship with the experience gives you more degrees of freedom in your attitude and in your actions in a given situation, whatever it is... even if you don't know what to do. The not knowing is its own kind of knowing, when the not knowing is itself embraced in awareness. Sounds strange, I know, but with ongoing practice, it may start making very real sense to you, viscerally, at a gut level, way deeper than thought.

Awareness transforms emotional pain just as it transforms the pain that we attribute more to the domain of body sensations. When we are immersed in emotional pain, if we pay close attention, we will notice that there is always an overlay of thoughts and a plethora of different feelings *about* the pain we are in, so here too the entire constellation of what we think of as emotional pain can be welcomed in and held in awareness, crazy as that may sound at first blush. It is amazing how unused we are to doing such a thing, and how profoundly revealing and liberating it can be to engage our emotions and feelings in this way, even when they are raging or despairing—especially when they are raging or despairing.

None of us need to inflict pain on ourselves just so we can have an occasion to test out this unique property of awareness to be bigger than and of a different nature altogether from our pain. All we need to do is be alert to the arrival of pain when it shows up, whatever its form. Our alertness gives rise to awareness at the moment of contact with the initiating event, whether it be a sensation or a thought, a look or a glance, what someone says, or what happens in any moment. The application of wisdom happens right here, *at* the point of contact, in the moment of contact (remember the princess who stubbed her toe?), whether you have just hit your thumb with a hammer or the world suddenly takes an unexpected turn and you are faced with one aspect or another of the full catastrophe, and all of a sudden grief and sorrow, anger and fear seem to have taken up what feels like permanent residency in your world.

It is at that moment, and in its aftermath, that we might bring awareness to the condition in which we find ourselves, the condition of the body and of the mind and heart. And then we take one more leap, bringing awareness to the awareness itself, noticing whether your awareness itself is in pain, or angry, or frightened, or sad.

It won't be. It can't be. But you have to check for yourself. There is no freedom in the thought of it. The thought is only useful in getting us to remember to look, to embrace that particular moment in awareness, and then to bring awareness to our awareness. That's when we check. You could even say that *is* the checking, because the awareness knows instantly. It may last only a moment, but in that moment lies the experience of freedom. The door to wisdom and heartfulness, the natural qualities of our being when we experience freedom, opens right in that moment. There is nothing else to do. Awareness opens it and invites you to peek in, if just for a second, and see for yourself.

This is not to suggest that awareness is a cold and unfeeling strategy for turning away from the depths of our pain in moments of anguish and loss or in their lingering aftermath. Loss and anguish, bereavement and grief, anxiety and despair, as well as all the joy available to us, lie at the very core of our humanity and beckon us to meet them face-on when they arise, and know them and accept them as they are. It is precisely a turning toward and an embracing, rather than a turning away or a denying or suppressing of feeling that is most called for and that awareness embodies. Awareness may not diminish the enormity of our pain in all circumstances. Nor should it. It does provide a greater basket for tenderly holding and intimately knowing our suffering in any and all circumstances, and that, it turns out, is transformative, and can make all the difference between endless imprisonment in pain and suffering and freedom from suffering, even though we have no immunity to the various forms of pain that, as human beings, we are invariably subject to.

Of course, opportunities large and small abound for bringing awareness to whatever is happening in our everyday lives, and so our whole life can become one seamless cultivation of mindfulness in this regard. Taking up the challenge of waking up to our lives and being transmuted by wakefulness itself is its own form of yoga, the yoga of everyday life, applicable in any and every moment: at work, in our relationships, in raising children if we are parents, in our relationships with our own parents whether they are living or dead, in our relationship with our own thoughts about the past and the future, in our relationship to our own bodies. We can bring awareness to whatever is happening, to moments of conflict and to moments of harmony, and to moments so neutral we might not notice them at all. In each moment, you can test out for yourself whether in bringing awareness to that moment, the world does or does not open in response to your gesture of mindfulness, does or does not "offer itself," in the poet Mary Oliver's lovely phrase, "to your imagination," whether or not it affords new and larger ways of seeing and being with what is, and thereby perhaps might liberate you from the dangers of partial seeing and the usually strong attachment you may have to any partial view simply because it is yours and you are therefore partial to it. Enthralled once again, even when in great pain, with the "story of me" that I am busy creating unwittingly, merely out of habit, I have an opportunity, countless opportunities, to see its unfolding and to cease and desist from feeding it, to issue a restraining order if necessary, to turn the key which has been sitting in the lock all along, to step out of jail, and therefore meet the world in new and more expansive and appropriate ways by embracing it fully rather than contracting, recoiling, or turning away. This willingness to embrace what is and then work with it takes great courage, and presence of mind.

So, in any moment, whatever is happening, we can always check and see for ourselves. Does awareness worry? Does awareness get lost in anger or greed or pain? Or does awareness brought to any moment, even the tiniest moment, simply know, and in knowing, free us? Check it out. It is my experience that awareness gives us back to ourselves. It is the only force I know that can do so. It is the quintessence of intelligence, physical, emotional, and moral. It seems as if it needs to be conjured up but in actuality, it is here all the time, only to be discovered, recovered, embraced, settled into. This is where the refining comes in, in remembering. And then, in the letting go and the letting be, resting in—in the words of the great Japanese poet Ryokan, "just this, just this." This is what is meant by the *practice* of mindfulness.

As we have seen, the challenge is twofold: first, to bring awareness to our moments as best we can, in even little and fleeting ways; second, to sustain our awareness and come to know it better and live inside its larger, never-ever-diminished wholeness. When we do, we see thoughts liberate themselves, even in the midst of sorrow, as when we reach out and touch a soap bubble. Puff. It is gone. We see sorrow liberate itself, even as we act to soothe it in others and rest in the poignancy of what is.

In this freedom, we can meet anything and everything with greater openness. We can hold the challenges we face now with greater fortitude, patience, and clarity. We already live in a bigger reality, one we can draw from by embracing pain and sorrow, when they arise, with wise and loving presence, with awareness, with uncontrived acts of kindness and respect toward ourself and toward others that no longer get lost in the illusory divide between inner and outer.

Yet to do so, to enact wakefulness, practically speaking, over the course of a lifetime, usually requires some kind of overarching framework that gives us a place to begin, recipes to try out, maps to follow, wise reminders to give ourselves, all the benefits to us of other people's hard-won experience and knowledge. And this would include, when we need them, various ramps into the awareness and freedom that are, ironically, here for us in any and every moment, and yet, at times, are seemingly so distant and far from our ken.

ON LINEAGE AND THE USES AND
LIMITATIONS OF SCAFFOLDING

If I have been able to see further, it was only because I stood on the shoulders of giants.

SIR ISAAC NEWTON

We all implicitly know that there is huge advantage to using what has come before, building on the creative genius and hard work of others who strained the limits of effort and dedication to see deeply into the nature of things, whether these forerunner explorers were scientists, poets, artists, philosophers, craftsmen, or yogis. In any domain that involves learning, we find ourselves standing on the shoulders of those who came before us and craning our necks to perceive what they, with huge dedication and effort, were able to discern. If we are wise, we will make every effort to read their maps, travel their roads, explore their methods, confirm their findings, so that we may know where to begin and what we might make our own, what to build upon, and where new insights, opportunities, and potential innovations lie. Often we are seriously oblivious of the ground we stand upon, the houses we live in, the lenses we see through, all gifted to us, mostly anonymously, by others. W. B. Yeats recognized our boundless debt to the creativity and labor of those who came before us and dedicated four lines of now immortal gratitude to those he called the unknown instructors, without whose profound yet in some ways fleeting, evanescent, and incomparable accomplishments, nothing further could be built or known:

What they undertook to do,
They brought to pass:
All things hang like a drop of dew
Upon a blade of grass.

Our ability to talk and think in words is one example of our inability to reach the heights of even our own innate biological capacity by our own efforts alone. We all have the potential for spoken language. But if a human being grows up in isolation from infancy, not learning language through exposure (either through hearing or through sign language), that capacity, it seems, cannot be fully developed later. Large swaths of mental functioning, cognitive and emotional, are arrested, and speech, even reasoning, severely curtailed.

The framework is here to begin with, but it needs to be primed, sculpted, shaped, nurtured through immersion in sounds made by humans, exposure to faces making those sounds, to eye contact, to inflection, to relationality with other humans, to their smells as well as their sounds, to a multimodal and richly sensory emotional connection. For the brain wires itself in important ways as a result of experiences. And this apparently needs to happen during a certain window of chronological development for language development to occur. If that window is somehow missed, we will remain mostly mute, with our own natural capacity and its potential flowering simply out of reach because the interpersonal, relational dimension was not there to hold and sculpt the innate capacity.

To take another, even more fundamental example, biology itself is utterly historical. New life only comes from old. Life builds on itself. Cells do not spring forth full-blown from noncellular environments, although it is thought that in the most rudimentary of forms they in all likelihood evolved originally within a prebiotic environment under vastly different conditions from those we have today, maybe three billion years ago. Cellular structure grows. It continually adds to itself, makes more of itself, while maintaining its own organizational integrity. This is called *autopoiesis*. Some scientists see it as the rudimentary first link between life and cognition, the original knowing of self if you will. Whether that is the case or not, we would not have new life without a preceding structure out of which it emerges seamlessly in its three-dimensional molecular architecture. Life is utterly historical.

Thus at every level—from the biological to the psychological to the social to the cultural—there is a fundamental need for what I call "scaffolding." We depend on instructions, guidelines, a context, a relationship, a language to venture meaningfully into the wilds of our own minds and the wilds of nature, the cosmos in which we find ourselves, even if we sometimes diverge from the beaten track and forge our own way through uncharted domains. That body of knowledge has been developed, refined, and distilled over centuries and millennia by lineages of those who have come before; lineages specializing in survival through hunting and gathering; lineages in the domestication of wild plants and animals; lineages in the sciences, in engineering and architecture, in the arts, and in the meditative traditions as well. These lineages have bequeathed to us a history of richly developed and hard-won knowledge of certain landscapes, and the skills required for navigating them effectively, distilled and framed in ways that we can build on, but only after we have penetrated and understood the paths others have blazed, their instructions for doing what they did and going where they went, only after we become intimate to at least some degree with the terrain and challenges they described and the solutions they arrived at.

This is our legacy in coming to meditation practice. For meditative practices did not arrive in our present era out of a vacuum. Those who came before us, the direct and multiply-branching lineages of teachers reaching back to the time of the Buddha and well before the Buddha, provide a road map, an offering, available for us to explore and take the measure of. These maps can amplify and enrich our possibilities for the inner exploration of the human mind and its potential that we have already embarked upon. As human beings, we are extraordinarily fortunate to have such a legacy available to us, to have such elevated and sturdy shoulders upon which to stand.

For, while the practices of meditation may seem at first blush fairly straightforward and perhaps even obviously beneficial, the full-scale power of meditative inquiry, the need for a rigorous discipline, the using of one's own life and mind and body as a laboratory for exploration of what is most fundamental to our humanness, the power inherent in a community of individuals who recognize their fundamental interconnectedness in a world of continual change and uncertainty and vulnerability, is a legacy we were not likely to come upon on our own, but one that, gifted to us more as a science of the mind and the heart than anything else, we can participate in and build upon, just as we individually and collectively build upon what came before in other domains of knowledge and understanding.

Of course, we know that there are rare, very rare instances of self-taught genius. But even Mozart studied with his father. Even the Buddha practiced in the meditative traditions of the day before charting his own path, beyond what he had learned from others, building on what had come before, inspired, as the story goes, merely by the sight of a wandering renunciate with a radiant and peaceful countenance who passed by him one day.

Almost all scientists themselves have mentors, or people who inspired them at one point or another to look and question deeply in perhaps a different and novel way. Even James Clerk Maxwell, who derived what are now known as Maxwell's equations of electromagnetism, one of the most colossal achievements in physics in the nineteenth century, anchored his efforts upon the work of Michael Faraday, who preceded him and shared many of his instincts, if not his mathematical virtuosity. To arrive at his breathtaking insight, describing precisely with four pristine equations the propagation of electromagnetic fields through space, Maxwell employed a mechanical analogy, a mental model of turning gears to explain to himself how these mysterious, never-before-visualized, incorporeal forces of electricity and magnetism might actually be related to each other. The model was entirely wrong, but it served him as a kind of scaffolding, allowing him to climb to where he was finally able to see, to reach a point where true insight into the nature of the forces he was attempting to understand was possible. The four equations he arrived at by climbing the thought-scaffold he erected were entirely correct and complete.

Maxwell was smart enough never to publish his mechanical model. He had transcended its utility. It had served its purpose. The lawfulness of invisible, intangible electromagnetic fields had been described with utter finality. The scaffolding was no longer important.

And so it is with meditation. We too can make good use of various kinds of scaffolding, much that we create for ourselves, much that we adopt from those who came before us, to both motivate us and assist us in coming to know and understand the terrain of our own minds and bodies and their intimately embedded relationship to the domain we call the world. Yet at a certain point, we will have to transcend the scaffolding, the platforms we have erected to help us to see, if we are to go beyond our own cognized and inherited models to the direct experiencing of what is being pointed to with instructions, words, and concepts.

Excluding rare exceptions, just sitting down for a time "to meditate" every once in a while or even regularly for years is not likely by itself to nurture insight, transformation, or liberation, even though that very impulse is priceless and the deep faith in one's own fundamental value and essential goodness is critical for undertaking that adventure. As a rule, we need to contextualize our efforts along these lines, yet without getting caught in the narratives that having such a framework and context usually entails.

Such meditation narratives would include the notion of a fixed destination. With meditation, clichéd as it may seem, as we have been intimating through our emphasis on the present moment and the realization that it is all already here and there is no "place" to go, it is the journey itself that is most important. The destination, in a very real way, is always "here," just as what is discoverable in science is always here even before it is seen, known, described, tested, confirmed, understood. Recall that Michelangelo claimed that he merely removed what needed removing from a block of marble, revealing the figure that he "saw" with his own deep artist's eye, that was, in a sense, there from the beginning. Yet without real work, whatever might be here to be revealed in the domains of our own minds and hearts, even though it is already here, remains opaque and of no use to us. It is only "here" in its potentiality. For it to be revealed requires us to participate in a process of possible revelation, and to be willing to be shaped and transmuted in turn by the process itself.

For this reason, it definitely helps to have a map of the terrain we will be entering when we begin meditating, while keeping very much in mind the important and deeply incisive reminder, although, again, some might say cliché, that the map is not the territory. The territory of the inner and outer landscapes of our experience as human beings and of our minds appears virtually limitless. Without a map to orient us in our meditation practice, we might very well wander in circles for days or decades without ever tasting moments of clarity or peace or freedom from our own oppressive ideas and opinions and desires. Without a map to orient us, we might also get easily caught by what was just said, perhaps idealizing the promise of a special outcome, caught up in illusions and self-deceptions about "getting somewhere," attaining clarity or peace or freedom, in the apparent paradox of it very much sounding like there really is some special place to get or state to attain. There is. And there isn't. That is why we need to have a map and why we need to follow the directions of those who have gone before, even while, or especially because, as we shall see further on in more detail, some of those very meditative directions are declaring that there is no map, there is no direction, no vision, no transformation, no attainment, and nothing to attain. Moreover, strange as it may sound, our motivation for practicing also needs to be entered into the equation, so that we don't go astray through an aggressive, acquisitive, striving attitude that is capable of unwittingly causing harm to ourselves or others along the way.

Confused at this point? Not a problem. Suffice it to say that you are likely to find it helpful to know something of the road you are treading and its vagaries, as reported by those who have traveled it in the past and mapped it out to whatever level of resolution they have managed in their own brief encounters with the infinite, just as it's a good idea to know how others have approached scaling Everest or any other mountain, rather than just going up trusting to luck and one's good intentions and judgment in the moment. It helps, no, it is critical to be equipped, outfitted, not merely with gear but with information and knowledge that come from the experience of others, with maps, and beyond that, to the degree that it is transferable, which it is not, but at least intuitable, it is essential to be equipped with your own innate but also informed wisdom. Otherwise, it is all too easy to delude oneself, and die needlessly on the mountain. It is hard enough to stay alive even with all the scaffolding to support you, and important that you not let it and all the details of getting there and surviving the journey prevent you from drinking in the fullness of the mountain's awesome beauty and presence, as well as your own, while you are there.

Even getting lost is not necessarily a problem. In fact, it may be an important part of the journey, and it can happen even when in possession of the best of maps. Getting lost and being confused, even making mistakes, are all an integral part of the learning. It is how we make the territory our own, how we come to know it intimately, firsthand.*

---

* For more on this subject, in the context of mindfulness and MBSR, see Kabat-Zinn, J. "Some Reflections on the Origins of MBSR, Skillful Means, and the Trouble with Maps." In Williams, J.M.G. and Kabat-Zinn, J. (Eds) *Mindfulness: Diverse Perspectives on Its Meaning, Origins, and Applications* (London: Routledge, 2013) 281–306.

*

Meditation practice invariably requires a certain kind of scaffolding, especially at the beginning (but really, always, to some degree, only it can grow to seem so second-nature that no "will" or "attempt" or "reminder" is any longer necessary), in the form of meditation instructions and a variety of methods and techniques. Such scaffolding also includes the larger context in which one would undertake such a strange lifelong adventure as to hone your own capacity for dwelling in stillness, for looking deeply into the nature of your own mind, and for realizing in this very moment and in all the moments that present themselves, the liberative dimensionality of awareness.

Just as we need scaffolding to build a building, just as scaffolding was needed for Michelangelo and his apprentices to paint the *frescos* on the ceiling of the Sistine Chapel, so we need a certain kind of framework to bring us to the essence of this inner work, right at the edge of this in-breath, this out-breath, this body, this moment.

But just as when the building is built or the ceiling completed, the scaffolding is no longer needed and comes down, never having been part of the essence of the endeavor, simply a necessary and useful means for furthering it, so with meditation, the very scaffolding of instructions and framework is dismantled, dismantles itself really, and only the impalpable, wordless essence remains, that essence being wakefulness itself, beyond and underneath, "before" thinking even arises.

What makes it interesting is that meditative scaffolding is needed in every moment, and by the same token, it needs to be dismantled in every moment, not later, at the end of some great work, such as the Sistine Chapel, but moment by moment. This is accomplished by knowing that it is merely scaffolding, however necessary and important, and not becoming attached to it. Letting it be erected and dismantled, moment by moment. With the Sistine Chapel, the scaffolding may need to be kept in storage, or resurrected for touching up, for restoration, for repair or fine-tuning over the years. But in the case of meditation, the masterpiece is always in progress and at the same time always complete in each moment, like life itself.

Put another way, proper instruction allows meditation to serve as the jumping-off point, right from the beginning, into what the Tibetans call *non-meditation*, even if it may only be a mysteriously opaque device at first, a mere suggestion to keep in mind for later. For *even the very thought that you are meditating is scaffolding*. That scaffolding is helpful in aiming and sustaining your practice, yet it is also important to see through it to actually be practicing. Both are operative simultaneously moment by moment as you sit, as you rest in awareness, as you practice in any way, beyond the reaches of the conceptual mind and its ceaseless proliferations and stories; even, or we could say, especially, your stories about meditation.

This very book, and all books on meditation, and all meditation teaching, lineages and traditions, however venerable, all CDs, downloads, apps, podcasts and other aids to practice are basically also really only scaffolding, or to switch images, fingers pointing at the moon, reminding us not only where to look but that there is something to behold, to see. We can fixate on the scaffolding or on the finger pointing, or refocus to directly apprehend what is being pointed to. The choice is always ours.

It is extremely important for us to know this and remember this from the very beginning of our encounter with meditation so as to not lose ourselves in or find ourselves clinging to the merely conceptual, to an ideal, or to a particular teacher or teaching or method or instruction, however enticing and satisfying any of that may appear to be. The risk of unawareness in this domain is that we might build up a convincing story about meditation and how important it is for us and fall into that narrative rather than realize the essence of who and what we actually are in the only moment we ever have to realize it, which is never some other moment.

ETHICS AND KARMA

Of course, even scaffolding needs a foundation upon which to rest. It is not very wise to erect it on shifting sands, or on dirt or clay that could easily turn into mud.

The foundation for mindfulness practice, for all meditative inquiry and exploration, lies in ethics and morality, and above all, in the motivation of non-harming. Why? Because you cannot possibly hope to know stillness and calmness within your own mind and body—to say nothing of perceiving the actuality of things beneath their surface appearances using your own mind as the instrument for knowing—or embody and enact those qualities in the world, if your actions are continually clouding, agitating, and destabilizing the very instrument through which you are looking, namely, your own mind.

We all know that when we transgress in some way, when we are dishonest, lie, steal, kill, cause harm to others, including through sexual misconduct, when we speak ill of people, when we stimulate, dull, or pollute our own minds by abusing substances such as alcohol and drugs out of our own unhappiness and desire for some relief from our pain, the consequences are invariably destructive, causing untold harm to others and to ourselves, whether we know it or not, whether we are beyond caring or not. Among the consequences of such actions is the certainty that they cloud the mind and fill it with various energies that prevent calmness, stability, and clarity, and the enlivened, deep-seeing perception that can accompany such clarity.

They take their toll on the body as well, tending to keep it chronically contracted, tense, aggressive, defensive, full of the effects of anger, fear, agitation, and confusion, and ultimately, isolation; and in all likelihood, also full of grief and remorse.

For this reason alone, it is important to examine how we are actually conducting our lives, what we are actually doing, what our actual behavior is, and to be aware of the downstream effects of our thoughts, words, and deeds, in the world and in our own hearts. If we are continually creating agitation in our lives, and causing harm to others and to ourselves, it is that agitation and harm that we will encounter in our meditation practice, because that is what we are feeding in ourselves. If we hope for a degree of peace in our own mind and heart, it is only commonsensical that we will benefit from no longer feeding those harmful tendencies and behaviors. In this way, just by forming the intention to recognize and back away from such impulses, we can begin to shift over from unhealthy, what Buddhists quaintly but accurately call "unwholesome," and destructive mind states and actions to healthier, more wholesome, and less clouded mind states and body states.

Generosity, trustworthiness, kindness, empathy, compassion, gratitude, joy in the good fortune of others, inclusiveness, acceptance and equanimity are qualities of mind and heart that further the possibilities of well-being and clarity within oneself, to say nothing of the beneficial effects they have in the world. They form the foundation for an ethical and moral life.

Greediness, attempting to take for oneself what is not freely given on any and every level, being untrustworthy and dishonest, unethical and immoral, cruel and full of ill will, riven and driven by self-centeredness at the expense of others, by anger and hatred, and lost in confusion, agitation, arrogance, and addiction, all these are qualities of mind that make it difficult to lead a life of inward satisfaction, equanimity, and peace—to say nothing of the harmful repercussions they have in the world. But mindfulness allows us to work with such mind states rather than merely deny them or suppress them, or continue to give vent to them. When we are visited by such energies, we can actually bring our awareness to them and, rather than be entirely consumed, examine them and learn from them about the sources of our suffering, feel and see the actual firsthand effects of our attitudes and actions on ourselves and on others, and experiment with the possibility of letting these very mind states become our meditation teachers and show us how to live and how not to live, where happiness lies, and where it is nowhere to be found.

What in the East is known as "karma" is basically the mystery of how our actions in the present wind up influencing what transpires downstream in time and space, for ourselves and for others. Whatever we have done in the past, the law of karma, of cause and effect, says that it will have inevitable consequences in the here and now, some subtle, some gross, some understandable, some not, some even imperceptible, all modulated by our original motivation and intention, the quality of mind that gave birth to the action itself. That can include, of course, as frequently happens, having no idea what our motivation was behind a particular thing that we did or said, because we were so caught up in the moment in an agitated state of mind, we literally didn't know what we were doing.

The past may be behind us, but we carry with us the accumulated consequences of what has already happened, whatever they may be, including perhaps remorse for past decisions and actions, or resentment for what happened to us that we were unable to prevent or control. Yet, with appropriate effort and appropriate support and scaffolding, we can also change our karma by coming to the present moment openly and mindfully as best we can, and forming the intention to shift from more afflictive and perhaps destructive to more nurturing mind states and body states. We change our karma in positive ways just by bringing awareness to our motivations, those underlying our outward actions, but also to those inward actions expressed in the mind and body through thoughts and through speech. By sustaining such an awareness of motivation over time, and by nurturing benevolent motivations and actively avoiding reacting reflexively out of unwholesome motives or total unawareness, in a word, by committing to and actually living an inwardly and outwardly ethical and moral life, moment by moment rather than just in principle, we prepare the ground for deep and ongoing transformation and healing. Without the ethical foundation, neither transformation nor healing is likely to take root. The mind will simply be too agitated, too caught up in its own unexamined conditioning, and in self-delusion and destructive emotions to provide appropriate soil for the cultivation of what is deepest, best, and healthiest in ourselves.

Ultimately, each one of us is morally, as well as usually legally, responsible for our own actions and their consequences. Recall that in adjudicating crimes against humanity, such as those perpetrated by the Nazis in World War II, or the My Lai massacre in Vietnam, or in Srebrenica, international war crimes tribunals have always found that ultimately, when all is said and done, the responsibility to preserve our humanity sits squarely on each one of us, no matter what our rank or status in society. There are times in which even in the military, disobeying orders takes precedence over obeying them. One reconnaissance helicopter pilot, Hugh Thompson Jr. flying over My Lai at the time of the massacre and seeing what was going on, landed his helicopter in the middle of the village and ordered his door gunners to fire on any of the American soldiers on the ground who continued to kill the women, children, and old men they were in the process of massacring. Ultimately, it is only individuals, each one of us, who can take a stand on the side of human goodness and kindness in the face of the immoral and the amoral and the unethical. Sometimes it may require the kind of dramatic action this 25-year old Army officer and his two crewmates took.* Sometimes it is entirely invisible, simply choosing to act ethically, even if you are the only person who will ever know. Or it may take the form of acts of civil disobedience for reasons of conscience, as when one chooses to publicly break a minor law

---

* For more detail on this remarkable incident, see Sapolsky, Robert M. *Behave: The Biology of Humans at Our Best and Worst*. (New York: Penguin, 2017) 656-658.

(and be willing to suffer the full legal consequences of one's actions) to bring attention to and to protest against actions or policies or laws within the body politic you consider to be immoral and harmful.

Both Gandhi and Martin Luther King Jr. used nonviolent civil disobedience to great effect in furthering the cause of human rights in the face of endemic and institutionalized cruelty and injustice. Such moral protesters are usually seen at the time by the government in power and often by many onlookers as troublemakers, as disrespectful of law and order, perhaps even as disloyal, unpatriotic, or even enemies of the state. But it could more accurately be said that they are patriots rather than enemies. They may be enemies only of injustice, marching to a different drummer, listening to and trusting the intelligence of their own conscience, voting with their feet and their bodies, their moral presence bearing witness to a larger truth. Notice that within a generation, they are usually revered, even sanctified.

But it is always harder to embody ethics and morality in the present moment, whoever one is, than to celebrate it in others, and usually only after they are long dead, and often murdered.

Ultimately ethics and morality are not about heroes and leaders and shining examples. They are about the day-to-day and moment-to-moment ways in which we conduct our own lives, and what our basic stance is toward those tendencies in our own minds that drive us toward greed, hatred, and delusion when what we most need is to tap the deeper resources of our own hearts for kindness, generosity, compassion, and goodwill. These are not merely sentimental feelings one might feel all cozy about on Christmas Eve, but truly a way to live, a practice in its own right, and the foundation of healing, transformation, and the possibilities available to us through meditation, and through mindfulness.

It is worth pointing out that, while it is a good idea for these issues to be raised in some fashion from the very beginning of meditation practice, it is also all too easy to fall into a kind of moralistic rhetoric that can sound a lot like sermonizing, and *that* invariably brings up legitimate questions in people's minds as to whether the person espousing such values actually adheres to them him- or herself, especially since there have been so many instances, including some in meditation centers, where those in positions of authority or power, whether religious figures, politicians, therapists, physicians, or lawyers, were breaking their own precepts and professional codes of ethics. Such codes of ethics may often be disregarded in the workplace, where rampant abuse of power is sometimes the norm, such as in the rampant sexual misconduct coming to light and finally being named by women regarding Hollywood moguls, movie stars, and television executives and pundits.

In the context of teaching MBSR in the Stress Reduction Clinic, we find it most effective and authentic to embody non-harming, openhearted presence, trustworthiness, generosity, and kindness as best we can as an essential part of our own practice, and in how we live and teach and carry ourselves, letting the more explicit conversations around morality and ethics arise naturally out of conversations in which people share in dialogue their experiences with the meditation practice itself, which means, with life itself. Attitudes of non-harming and the clear seeing of reactive and destructive mind states and habits are an intimate part of the meditation instructions themselves, and attending carefully to them as we practice together tends to entrain all of us into greater awareness of the benefits of certain thought streams and actions, and the dangers of others, including unawareness of power differentials, tacit and unacknowledged assumptions about others, and unrecognized privilege.

Ethics and morality are seen, known, and recognized through being lived far more than they are through words, however eloquent. And in a way, as you will undoubtedly see and feel and experience for yourself, they are inherent in the cultivation of mindfulness, by seeing and feeling firsthand (in other words recognizing for ourselves) the inner and outer effects of our actions, our words, and even our thoughts, our emotions, and our facial expressions, whatever they may be, literally moment by moment, breath by breath, and day by day.

MINDFULNESS

So, after all this talk of mindfulness, what is it really anyway?

According to the Buddhist scholar and monk Nyanaponika Thera, mindfulness is

> the unfailing master key for *knowing* the mind and is thus the starting point; the perfect tool for *shaping* the mind, and is thus the focal point; and the lofty manifestation of the achieved *freedom* of the mind, and is thus the culminating point.

Not bad for something that basically boils down to paying attention and being awake.

Mindfulness can be thought of as moment-to-moment, non-judgmental awareness, cultivated by paying attention in a specific way, that is, in the present moment and as non-reactively, as non-judgmentally, and as openheartedly as possible. The non-judgmental part doesn't mean that you won't have any judgments! On the contrary, it means that you will discover that you have tons of judgments, but that you will be more inclined to recognize them for what they are, namely preferences of all kinds, judgments, liking, disliking, desire, aversion. Being non-judgmental is thus an invitation to intentionally suspend the judging as best you can, while noticing how much it goes on.

When it is cultivated intentionally, mindfulness is sometimes referred to as *deliberate mindfulness*. When it spontaneously arises, as it tends to do more and more the more it is cultivated intentionally, it is sometimes referred to as *effortless mindfulness*. Ultimately, however arrived at, mindfulness is mindfulness. It is wakefulness, pure and simple. It is awareness. It is open-hearted presence.

Of all the meditative wisdom practices that have developed in traditional cultures throughout the world and throughout history, mindfulness is perhaps the most basic, the most powerful, the most universal, among the easiest to grasp and engage in, and arguably, the most sorely needed now. For mindfulness is none other than the capacity we all already have to know what is actually happening as it is happening. Vipassana teacher Joseph Goldstein describes it as that "quality of mind that notices what is present without judgment, without interference. It is like a mirror that clearly reflects what comes before it." Larry Rosenberg, another vipassana teacher, calls it "the observing power of the mind, a power that varies with the maturity of the practitioner." But, we might add, if mindfulness is a mirror, it is a mirror that knows *non-conceptually* what comes within its scope. And, not being two-dimensional, we might say that it is more like an electromagnetic or gravitational field than a mirror, a field of knowing, a field of awareness, a field of emptiness, in the same way that a mirror is intrinsically empty, and can therefore "contain" anything and everything that comes before it. Awareness is boundless, or at least it feels that way inwardly, boundless like space itself, with no center and no periphery.

If mindfulness is an innate quality of mind, it is also one that can be refined through systematic practice. And for most of us, it *has* to be refined through practice. We have already noted how out of shape we tend to be when it comes to exercising our innate capacity to pay attention. And that is what meditation is all about...the systematic and intentional cultivation of mindful presence, and through it, of discernment, wisdom, compassion, and other qualities of mind and heart conducive to breaking free from the fetters of our own persistent blindness, self-centeredness, and delusions.

The attentional stance we are calling mindfulness has been described by Nyanaponika Thera as "the heart of Buddhist meditation." It is central to all the Buddha's teachings and to all the Buddhist traditions, from the many currents and streams of Zen in China, Korea, Japan, and Vietnam, to the various schools of vipassana or "insight meditation" in the Theravada tradition native to Burma, Cambodia, Thailand, and Sri Lanka, to those of Tibetan (Vajrayana) Buddhism in India, Tibet, Nepal, Ladakh, Bhutan, Mongolia, and Russia. And now, virtually all of these schools and their attendant traditions have established firm roots in the cultures of the West, where they are presently flourishing.

Their relatively recent arrival in the West over the past two generations or so is a remarkable historical extension of a flowering that emerged out of India in the centuries following the death of the Buddha and ultimately spread across Asia in these many forms and also returned relatively recently to India, where it had fallen into decline for hundreds of years.

Strictly speaking, from an instrumental perspective, the cultivation of mindfulness provides reliable access to our innate awareness. What we are refining is *access* to awareness rather than awareness itself. The more we can attend moment by moment and non-judgmentally, the more we can dwell in awareness itself, be the wakefulness of awareness. At the same time, from a non-instrumental perspective, mindfulness and awareness are already identical. No development is necessary. Paradoxically, we already have what we are seeking or hoping to cultivate. All that is required is to get out of our own way, which ironically often takes some work. In what follows, we will be using the words mindfulness and awareness synonymously, recognizing that the instrumental and the non-instrumental are themselves not separate but complementary interpenetrating aspects of a larger wholeness.

What is more, since there is nothing particularly Buddhist about paying attention or about awareness, the essence of mindfulness both as a practice and as synonymous with awareness itself is truly universal. It has more to do with the nature of the human mind than with any ideology, beliefs, or culture. It has more to do with our capacity for knowing (as we have already observed, what is called *sentience*) than with a particular religion, philosophy, or view. Ultimately, mindfulness is a way of being. It is not a technique, a philosophy, or a catechism.

Returning to the simile of the mirror, it is the cardinal virtue of any mirror, small or large, that it can contain any landscape, depending on how it is turned and whether it is clear or covered with dust or dulled by age. There is no necessity to anchor the mirror of mindfulness and restrict it to one particular view to the exclusion of other equally valid inner and outer landscapes. There are many ways of knowing. Mindfulness subsumes and includes them all, just as we might say there is one truth, not many, but there are many ways in which it is understood and can be expressed in the vastness of time and space and the plenitude of cultural conditions and locales.

Yet the mirror is a limited simile or metaphor for mindfulness in other ways, even though it is exceedingly useful at times. For not just is it two dimensional; it is also a reflected image, and thus always reversed. When you look at your face in the mirror, it is not your face as it is seen by the world, but the mirror image of it, where left is right and right is left. Being a surface, it does not reflect things quite as they actually are but renders merely an illusion of such.

Mindfulness is valued, perhaps not by that name, but by its qualities, in virtually all contemporary and ancient cultures. Indeed, one might say that our lives and our very presence here have depended on the clarity of the mind as mirror and its refined capacity to reflect, contain, encounter, and know with great fidelity things as they actually are. For example, our early ancestors needed to make instant and correct assessments of situations virtually moment by moment. In any moment, their ability to do that well could spell the difference between survival of an individual or even a whole community, and extinction. Thus every person now on Earth is the progeny exclusively of generations of survivors. There was clearly an evolutionary advantage to a mind that could mind what was happening in real time and know instantly that what it knew could be relied upon and acted on. Those whose mirrors were perhaps somewhat flawed may not have made decisions that effectively insured their survival long enough to pass on their genes. In this way, there was definite selective advantage to clear mirrors that could instantly recognize and reflect accurately in any matter impinging on survival all the messages coming through the sense doors.

We are the inheritors of that perpetually self-refining selection process. In that sense, we are all above average. Far above average. Miraculous beings really, when you stop and think about it.

Over the centuries, the universal inborn capacity we all have for exquisitely fine-tuned awareness and insight has been explored, mapped, preserved, developed, and refined—not so much anymore by prehistory's hunting-and-gathering societies, which sadly, along with everything they know of the world, are on the verge of extinction brought on by the "successes" of the flow of human history, such as agriculture and the division and specialization of labor and the rise cities and of ever-advancing technologies—but rather in monasteries. These intentionally sequestered environments sprang up early in antiquity and have weathered millennia of vicissitudes, all the while renouncing worldly concerns to better devote their energies solely to cultivating, refining, and deepening mindfulness and putting it to use to investigate the nature of the mind with the intention to come to a full and embodied realization of what it means to be fully human and become free from the prison of habitual mental affliction and suffering. At their best, these monasteries were veritable laboratories for investigating the mind, and the monastics who populated them and continue to do so to this day used themselves as both the scientists and the object of study in these ongoing investigations.

These monks and nuns and occasional householders took for their North Star the example of the Buddha and his teachings. The Buddha, as we have seen, was a person who, for various karmic reasons, took it upon himself to sit down and direct his attention to the central question of suffering, to the investigation of the nature of the mind itself, and to the potential for liberation from sickness, old age, and death, and from what might be called the fundamental dis-ease of humanity. He did this not by denying any of these domains or attempting to circumvent them. Rather, he did it by looking directly into the nature of human experience itself, using as his instrument the capacity we all share but hardly ever refine to such an extent, for looking into anything in the first place, namely, unwavering attention and the awareness and potential for deep and clarifying insight that stem from it. He described himself, when asked, not as a god, as some would have had it, awed by his wisdom, apparent luminosity, and mere presence, but simply as "awake." That wakefulness followed directly from his experience of seeing deeply into the human condition and human suffering and his discovery that it was possible to break out of seemingly endless cycles of self-delusion, misperception, and mental affliction to an innate freedom, equanimity, and wisdom.

Throughout our work together in this volume and the following ones, we will be coming back to mindfulness over and over again, to what it is and to the different ways, both formal and informal, it can be cultivated, all the while hopefully not getting caught in our stories about it, even as we unavoidably generate them. We will examine mindfulness from many different angles, feeling our way into its various energies and properties, and how they may be relevant to the specifics of our everyday lives on every level, and to our short- and long-term well-being and happiness.

We will start by taking a closer look at why paying attention is so critically important to our well-being in the first place, and how it fits into the larger scheme of healing and transforming both our lives and the world.

PART 2

THE POWER OF ATTENTION
AND THE DIS-EASE OF THE WORLD

———

The faculty of voluntarily bringing back a wandering attention,
over and over again, is the very root of judgment, character, and will.
No one is compos sui *if he have it not.*
An education which should improve this faculty
would be the education par excellence.
But it is easier to define this ideal
than to give practical instructions for bringing it about.

WILLIAM JAMES, *Principles of Psychology* (1890)

Why Paying Attention Is So Supremely Important

William James obviously didn't know about the practice of mindfulness when he penned the passage on the preceding page, but I am sure he would have been delighted to have discovered that there was indeed an education for improving the faculty of voluntarily bringing back a wandering attention over and over again. For this is precisely what Buddhist practitioners have developed into a fine art over millennia, based on the Buddha's original teachings, and this art is replete with practical instructions for bringing this kind of self-education about. While James was bemoaning the absence of something that already existed at that time in a universe half-way round the world that was unavailable to him, the founder of modern American psychology nevertheless clearly put his finger on the magnitude of the problem. He understood how endemically the mind wanders, and how critically important it is to ride herd on one's own attention if one hopes to live fully a life of, as he put it, "judgment, character, and will."

For, paying attention is something we do so selectively and haphazardly that we often don't see what is right in front of our eyes or even hear sounds that are carried to us through the air and are clearly entering our ears. The same can be said for our other senses as well. Perhaps you've noticed it in yourself.

It is easy to eat without tasting, miss the fragrance of the moist earth after a rain, even touch others without knowing the feelings we are transmitting. In fact, we refer to all these ever-so-common instances of missing what is here to be sensed, whether they involve our eyes, our ears, or our other senses, as examples of being *out of touch*.

We use touch as a metaphor for relating through all the senses because, in fact, we are literally touched by the world through all our senses, through our eyes, ears, nose, tongue, body, and also through our mind.

For all that, we tend to be specialists at being out of touch a great deal of the time, and out of touch with just how out of touch we can be.

If we examine this phenomenon by simply observing our interior and exterior lives from time to time, it soon becomes quite apparent just how much of the time we are out of touch. We are out of touch with our feelings and perceptions, with our impulses and our emotions, with our thoughts, with what we are saying, and even with our bodies. This is mostly due to being perpetually preoccupied, lost in our minds, absorbed in our thoughts, obsessed with the past or the future, consumed with our plans and desires, diverted by our need to be entertained, driven by our expectations, fears, or cravings of the moment, however unconscious and habitual all this may be. And therefore, we can be and usually are amazingly out of touch in one way or other with the present moment, the moment that is actually presenting itself to us now.

And our out-of-touchness is not limited to not seeing things that are right in front of us, or not hearing what is clearly coming to our ears, or missing out on the world of fragrance and taste and touch because we are so preoccupied and distracted. How many times have you unwittingly and improbably walked into the door you were opening, or inadvertently banged your hand or elbow on something, or dropped something you didn't know you were carrying because in that moment, you weren't actually all there, and so were momentarily out of touch even with the spatial and temporal orientation of the body, which normally we have covered without too much specific attention?

And is it not the case that we are sometimes equally and grossly out of touch with what we call the "outside" world, with our effects on other people, with what they care about and may be going through and feeling, even when it is written on their faces or apparent in their body language, if only we were available to ourselves to take notice?

Yet, the only way we can be in touch with any of this is through our senses. They are the only ways we have of knowing either the interior world of our own being, or the outer landscape we call "the world."

We have more senses than we think. Intuition is a kind of sense. Proprioception—the body knowing how it is positioned in space—is a sense. Interoception—the overall interior *feel* of the body as a whole— is a sense. The mind itself can also be thought of as a sense, and indeed, as already noted, it is characterized as the sixth sense door in Buddhist teachings. For most of what we feel and know of both the inner landscape and the outer landscape completes itself through processing within the mind. Without mind, even our perfectly intact senses of eyes, ears, nose, tongue, and skin would not give us a very useful picture of the world we inhabit. We need to know what we are seeing, hearing, tasting, smelling, touching, and we know it only through the interaction between the sense itself and what we call mind, that mysterious knowing quality of sentience or consciousness that includes thought but is not limited merely to thought. So we could accurately call awareness itself our sixth sense rather than mind. In a way, awareness and mind essence are two ways of saying the same thing.

Much of what we actually know, we know in a non-conceptual way. Thinking and memory come in a bit later, but very quickly, on the heels of an initial moment of pure sense contact. Thinking and memory can easily color our original experience in ways that distort or detract from the bare experience itself. That is why painters so often prefer to feel their way into a new painting rather than to have it merely come out of the conceptual. The conceptual has its place, but it often follows and only informs those raw feelings that move the senses to awaken in fresh and surprising ways. Bare perception is raw, elemental, vital, and thus, creative, imaginative, revealing. With our senses intact and by way of awareness itself, we can attend in such ways. To do so is to be more alive.

> *Now what shall we call this new form of gazing-house*
> *that has opened in our town where people sit*
> *quietly and pour out their glancing*
> *like light, like answering?*

> RUMI, "NO ROOM FOR FORM"
> *Translated by Coleman Barks with John Moyne*

*

In teaching about the importance of attention in health and well-being, I have found it useful and illuminating to feature a model first articulated by psychologist Gary Schwartz that emphasizes attention's pivotal role in health and disease. Consider the effects of not paying attention to what our bodies and minds are constantly telling us. For long stretches of time, of course, especially if we are fairly healthy to begin with, we can get away with not paying attention to anything. Or at least it seems that way on the surface. But if various signs and symptoms, even subtle ones, are ignored, left unattended for too long, and if the condition you find yourself in is too much of a burden on the body or the mind, this *dis-attention* can lead to *dis-connection*, the atrophying or disruption of specific pathways whose finely tuned integrity is necessary to maintain the dynamic processes that underlie health. This dis-connection can in turn lead to *dis-regulation*, where things actually start to go wrong, swing grossly away from the natural homeostatic balance. Dis-regulation in turn can lead to outright *dis-order* on the cellular, tissue, organ, or systems level, a breakdown into dis-regulated, chaotic processes. This dis-order in turn leads to or manifests as outright *disease*, or put otherwise, to *dis-ease*.

We could take virtually any condition as a case in point because the approach applies in any and all circumstances. But to keep it simple, let's take as an example not paying attention to, say, neck pain that might first appear as sensations of stiffness or muscle tightness. That would be the first sign, or indication, especially if it persisted, of something that needed attending to, either in the form of seeing a doctor or beginning a physical therapy or yoga program, or both. Ignored, it might gradually become more frequent and severe, turning into a chronic complaint, a symptom perhaps of something deeper going on. By that time, we might have gotten kind of used to it, and if the pain is not too bad, and if we are very busy, we might just write it off to tension or stress, and continue to ignore it. Over weeks, months, even years, if not attended to, such a condition will either go away on its own, or tend to worsen, especially in response to stress, and it might make us more prone to injury, say if we turn our head too quickly while driving, or even lie in bed the wrong way. By that time, it may have become something of a syndrome that we have gotten so used to that we have learned to ignore it completely or tolerate it, perhaps denying the potential importance of doing something about it. This disconnection on our part can lead to a gradual disregulation of the muscles and nerves in the neck in the form of chronic tension and even postural compensations that, in turn, can affect the bones and connective tissue over time to compound the condition. Things can get disregulated to the point where our neck no longer functions normally, and the pain and discomfort and physical limitations in range of motion and posture worsen. This in turn can predispose us to inflammation in response to irritation or injury, a further disordering of things, followed perhaps by an increased likeliness of arthritis, a more serious disease condition that brings with it a great deal of dis-ease or discomfort.

By the same token, we can say that *attention*, and in particular, wise attention, not neurotic self-preoccupation and hypochondriasis, reestablishes and strengthens *connection* or connectedness. Connection in turn leads to greater *regulation*, which leads to a state of dynamic *order*, which is the signature of *ease*, of well-being, of health, as opposed to disease. And for this to take place, of course, attention has to be maintained and nourished by *intention*, so attention and intention together play an intimate role in supporting each other, the yin and the yang underlying health and healing, as well as clarity and compassion.

In the above example, paying attention might involve taking care of our neck by going to a yoga class, or getting a good massage from time to time, or training ourselves to notice how stress and tension can accumulate in the neck at particular times and how even our aware-ness of it can influence and perhaps minimize those occurrences. We literally and metaphorically become more in touch with the neck, what it is up to, and what it is capable of. This connectivity leads to greater regulation, as the neck responds to our attention. Continued attention to the body's messages might be furthered additionally by taking an MBSR program to learn how to deal with accumulated ten-sion in our life so that it doesn't always wind up in our neck (literally becoming "a pain in the neck"), perhaps learning something as simple as bringing greater mindfulness to the sensations in the neck so that we are in touch with those early warning signs and symptoms and can recognize them rather than ignore them, and perhaps learn how to let the breath dispel some of the accumulated tension. In this way, the concatenation of circumstances predisposing us to a worsening of the condition may be nipped in the bud, and we continue to experience increasing "order" and ease and an absence of neck pain, even under stress, rather than ever-increasing neck problems.

However, it is always possible when we pay close attention to something that we will at times fall unwittingly into mis-perception, when for whatever reason, we do not see clearly what is unfolding in a particular moment, and thereby miss the real connection and the chain leading up from attention to greater connection and ulti-mately, to ease, and thus to health, clarity, even a degree of wisdom (in relationship to the neck) and compassion (in being more kind to yourself and your neck). That moment of mis-perception can itself, if unattended to, lead to a mis-apprehension, a mis-appraisal of a situation or circumstance, and from there to a possible mis-attribution of its particular cause.

That in turn can lead to an outright and literal mis-take, a mis-taking of what we think to be true for the actuality of how things are, followed by acting on that causal chain from *mis-perception* to *mis-apprehension*, to *mis-appraisal*, to *mis-attribution*, to *mis-take*. It happens in our daily lives in those moments when we actually make mistakes, mistakes usually caused by mis-perception and mis-attribution. If unexamined, this can be a parallel route to dis-ease, psychologically, socially, and physically.

In our example of the neck pain, a mis-perception might take the form of an obsessive preoccupation with fleeting sensations in the neck that we might exaggerate into pain, making a mountain out of a molehill, so to speak, leading to hypochondriasis and maybe even wearing a neck brace unnecessarily, while not exercising the neck in ways that could make it stronger and more flexible. We might be walking around identifying with what we tell ourselves is a chronic neck problem, and missing all opportunities for looking more deeply into it. We could call this a form of *unwise attention*, rooted in a reactive self-preoccupation that keeps us stuck in disconnection of a different order.

Such unwise attention also drives things all too frequently at the level of the body politic, when people are stampeded into formulating new policies or making decisions on the basis of wrong, incomplete, or mis-analyzed information, or driven by underlying motives, often unexamined, which put personal self-interest above the wisdom of considering the well-being of the whole and how to further it. The consequences of such mis-perceptions and mis-takes can be non-trivial, resulting in missed opportunities of all sorts. Often such mis-takes can lead unnecessarily to the inflaming of already incendiary situations that could have been perceived more accurately in the first place, were the lenses of perception and their state of clarity or lack of clarity objects of attention at the beginning. For such reasons, accurate perception and correct apprehension are key elements in our ability to come to our senses, literally and metaphorically.

When, through the practice of mindfulness, we learn to listen to the body through all its sense doors, as well as to attend to the flow of our thoughts and feelings, we are beginning the process of reestablishing and strengthening connectedness within our own inner landscape. That attention nurtures a familiarity and an intimacy with our lives unfolding at the level of what we call body and what we call mind that deepens and strengthens well-being and a sense of ease in our relationship to whatever is unfolding in our lives from moment to moment. We thus move from dis-ease, including outright disease, to greater ease and harmony and, as we shall see, greater health.

And this is as true, as we shall come to examine further on, for our institutions and for the body politic as it is for the body and for our individual minds.

Dis-Ease

Consume my heart away; sick with desire
And fastened to a dying animal
It knows not what it is, . . .

W. B. Yeats, "Sailing to Byzantium"

With regard to disease and dis-ease, we might say that the most fundamental dis-ease stemming from disattention and disconnection, and from mis-perception and mis-attribution, is the anguish of the human condition itself, of the full catastrophe unmet and unexamined.

As suggested by the opening sentence of our meditation brochure for business leaders, which speaks of the unexamined whispered longings of the heart, virtually everybody has to some degree or other whispered longings from deep within the psyche, a secret life really, a life full of dreams and possibilities we usually keep hidden. The sad thing is, we usually keep it hidden from ourselves too. We suffer greatly as a consequence. The secret is sustained often for the whole of our lives with no inkling that we are complicit in a self-deception that can be severely life-eroding and self-destructive.

The real secret? That we really do not know who or what we are, for all the surface preoccupations, pretensions, and the inward and outward posturing we construct and hide behind to keep ourselves and everybody else in the dark.

For are not our hearts at various times filled with, driven, even tormented by unsatisfied and seemingly endless desires, great and small, no matter how outwardly successful and comfortable we may appear to be? And are we not vaguely aware on some subterranean level of the psyche that we are indeed "fastened" to a dying animal? And that we do not know who and what we actually are?

In three lines, Yeats captures three fundamental aspects of the human condition: one, that we are unfulfilled and suffer for it; two, that we are subject to sickness, old age, and death, the inexorable law of impermanence and constant change; and three, that we are ignorant of the true nature of our very being.

Isn't it time for us to discover that we are already larger than we allow ourselves to know? Isn't it time for us to discover that it is possible to inhabit that larger knowing and perhaps free ourselves from the deep anguish of our persistent habit of ignoring what is most important? I would argue that it is long past time, and that now is also the perfect time.

True, we may feel at times intimations of our discomfort in vague stirrings within the psyche. Once in a rare while, we may even catch momentary glimpses of it waking up disoriented and frightened in the middle of the night, or when someone close to us suffers deeply or dies, or our own life's framework suddenly unravels as if it had always been primarily in some strange way merely imagined. But then, isn't it true that as soon as possible, we go back to sleep literally and metaphorically, and anesthetize ourselves with one diversion or another?

This primordial human dis-ease of which Yeats speaks, that we know not what we are, feels too huge to bear. Thus, we bury it deep within the psyche, secreted away, well sequestered from daylight consciousness. Often, as we have seen, it takes an acute crisis to awaken us to it, and to the possibilities of true healing and freeing ourselves from the darkness of our fear and our ignoring.

We suffer greatly in body and mind from this turning away from these deepest intimations of our humanity. We may feel consumed, to use Yeats's word, literally "eaten up," and also diminished in countless ways because we neglect the full reality of what we are. Yet we might not know that with any clarity or conviction either.

This dis-ease of unawareness, of ignoring what is most fundamental in our own nature as beings, affects our lives as individuals virtually from moment to moment, and over the course of decades. It can produce short- and long-term effects on our health of both body and mind. It cannot help but color family life and work life in ways that often remain unseen, or that are not discovered until years after certain kinds of damage have been done and unwise roads unwittingly pursued. And its presence spills out to influence society through our collective ways of seeing ourselves and of doing business. It pervades our institutions and the ways we shape or ignore our inner and outer environments.

Everything we do is colored in one way or another by our ignoring the malaise of not knowing who we are and how we are. It is the ultimate affliction, the ultimate disease. And as such, it gives rise to many variants, to many different manifestations of anguish and suffering at the level of the body, the mind, and the world.

DUKKHA

Buddhists have a remarkable and extremely useful word for the dis-ease stemming from being filled with desire, fastened to a dying animal, and not knowing what we are.

They call it *dukkha*, a Pali term in the language in which the Buddha's teachings were first written down. The meaning of *dukkha* is exceedingly difficult to capture in one English word. It is rendered variously by translators and scholars as *suffering, anguish, stress, malaise, dis-ease,* or *unsatisfactoriness.*

The first Noble Truth of the Buddha's teachings is the centrality, universality, and unavoidability of dukkha, the innate suffering of dis-ease that invariably, in subtle or not-subtle-at-all ways, colors and conditions the deep structure of our very lives. All Buddhist meditative practices revolve around the recognition of dukkha, the identification of its root causes, and the description, development, and deployment of pathways whereby we might each become free from its oppressive, blinding, and imprisoning influences. These pathways to freedom from suffering, from dukkha, are all one pathway really, a method aimed at awakening us to what we have been keeping secret or hidden from ourselves. How? By paying wise attention to whatever arises in our experience instead of what we usually tend to do, which is either not to pay attention to it at all, or alternatively, to wallow in it, romanticize it, quietly and hopelessly endure it, struggle against it, downright drown in it, or endlessly distract ourselves to escape from it.

Such a pathway offers the possibility of leading a far more satisfying and authentic life. So the truth of the universality of dukkha is actually not some maudlin and passive bemoaning of its inevitability—precisely because this dissatisfaction and sometimes anguish is neither enduring nor intrinsically limiting. It can be worked with, even in its most horrific aspects. It can become our teacher. It can serve to show us how we can free ourselves from its grasp.

And importantly, our exploration of the possibility of liberation from suffering, from dukkha, and the living of a more authentic and satisfying life is not undertaken merely for ourselves—although that in itself would be quite an accomplishment and may be the proximal motivation that brings us to mindfulness practice—but in very real and nonromantic ways, for the benefit of all beings with whom our lives are inexorably entwined. It turns out that that is a lot of beings, the whole universe really.

Lying at the heart of all these meditative practices for the recognition of, liberation from, and cessation of dukkha is the cultivation of mindfulness, an entirely different way of relating to this pervasive condition of dis-ease, one that involves embracing it and being willing to work with it, to observe it without bias in its most intimate characteristics. As we have said, mindfulness can be thought of as an openhearted, non-judgmental, present-moment awareness, the direct, non-conceptual knowing of experience as it unfolds, in its arising, in its momentary lingering, and in its passing away. Addressing those dedicated to the embodiment of his teachings through intensive and systematic practice, the Buddha said:

this is the direct path for the purification of beings,
for the surmounting of sorrow and lamentation,
for the disappearance of pain and grief,
for the attainment of the true way,
for the realization of liberation—
namely, the four foundations of mindfulness.

Quite an assertion.

All of Buddhism is oriented toward waking up from the delusions we spin for ourselves and the ones we are conditioned into through past experiences. In awakening, we free ourselves from the suffering and anguish that come from mis-taking the nature of reality through our limited self-oriented views and tendency to grasp and cling to what we desire and to push away what we fear.

In the past twenty-six hundred years, the various meditative traditions within Buddhism have developed, explored, and refined a range of highly sophisticated and effective methods for the cultivation of mindfulness and of the wisdom and compassion that emerge naturally from its practice. There are many doors into the room of mindfulness. While the view from each one might be quite different in some respects, the important thing is to enter the room. The door to choose is the one that is most congenial to you, or the most convenient, for whatever reason. But above all, the invitation is to enter, enter, enter, rather than stand in the doorway and comment about it.

Just as it has been argued by Thomas Cahill that the Irish saved Western civilization by the copying of ancient manuscripts by monastics during the Middle Ages in Europe, and the gift of the Jews was to give the world its first articulation of historical time unfolding and therefore a sense of the possibility of the development of the individual within time, in personal connection with the numinous, so we could say that the historical figure of the Buddha and those who have followed his lead gave the world a well-defined algorithm, a path of inquiry, which he himself pursued in search of what was most fundamental to the nature of humanity: the possibility of being fully conscious, fully awake, and free from the fetters of our own conditioning, including our unexamined habits of thought and perception and the afflictive emotions that so intimately and frequently accompany them unbidden.

DUKKHA MAGNETS

Consider this. Whether you want to call it stress or dis-ease or dukkha, it is pretty obvious that hospitals function as major dukkha magnets in our society. Their force fields pull in those among us who are suffering the most at any given moment either from disease or dis-ease or both; from stress, pain, trauma, and illness of all kinds. People go or are taken to the hospital when there is literally nowhere else to go, when they have run out of other options and resources. As a rule, hospitals are not places we go to have fun or to be entertained or enlightened. But they are very much the places we go when we seek to be treated and hopefully repaired and fixed (we say "fixed up") if not cured. We go with the expectation that we will be met and met adequately, met appropriately, and that we will be tended to with care and attention; and if we are very fortunate, perhaps "enlightened" as to what is going on with us and what we need to do.

Given the level of suffering hospitals attract, one might think, "What better place to offer training in mindfulness, said by no less an authority than the Buddha himself to be the direct path for the surmounting of sorrow and lamentation and the disappearance of pain and grief, in a word, the relief of suffering? Might not some exposure to mindfulness, if it is indeed as powerful and as fundamental and as universal as the Buddha was claiming, be of significant benefit to many of the people who walk or are carried through its doors?" Of course, such an offering would be available not as a substitute for good and compassionate medical care, but as a potentially vital complement to whatever treatments they might be receiving. And what better place to offer such training, not only for the patients but for the staff as well, who in many instances are just as stressed as the patients?

This is how mindfulness-based stress reduction (MBSR) came to be born. At first it was offered primarily for those medical patients who could be said to be falling through the cracks of the health care system, people who were not being completely helped by the medical treatments available to them. That turned out to be a lot of people. It also included a great many people who had not improved with traditional medical treatment or were suffering from intractable conditions for which medicine has few options and no cures. And we were happy to be able to offer them an opportunity to explore the boundaries of the possible for themselves.

However, the program soon attracted an even broader spectrum of patients within the hospital. After all, "stress reduction" has an innate appeal. The almost universal response to the signs in the corridors pointing to Stress Reduction is "I could use that," followed, of course, in many cases, by "But of course, I don't have the time for it." But at this juncture, almost forty years after it started, more and more patients and even more and more physicians are realizing that they may not be able to afford *not* to take the program and begin paying more careful attention to what has for so long been unattended.

From its inception, MBSR gave physicians across a wide range of disciplines and specialties a new option for their patients. The Stress Reduction Clinic was a place within the hospital where medical patients could, on an outpatient basis, learn to do something for themselves as a complement to all the treatments and procedures that were being done for or to them, something potentially extremely powerful and also hard to come by, precious.

In parallel, the option to refer their patients to MBSR also gave physicians a way to relieve their own stress stemming from the patients for whom they no longer had good treatment options but who kept coming back with their complaints and, in many cases, were majorly dissatisfied with their treatments or lack of them. Now there was a place to send them within the hospital where, within a highly structured, supportive, and emotionally safe environment, they could be invited to take on a higher degree of responsibility for their own experience and the states of mind and body they were experiencing and suffering from, however painful, problematic, or chronic those conditions were; a program that would offer them and guide them in the possibility of tapping into hitherto unknown but very deep and universal inner resources at their disposal for learning, growing, healing, and transformation, not just for the eight weeks that they were in the program, but hopefully for the rest of their lives.

In the process, people who had felt to a large degree like passive recipients of health care would have an opportunity to become full participants and vital partners in their own ongoing health care and well-being. And they would be able to undergo such a process while being fully seen and met and held in high regard by the class instructor simply for being human and for being who they were and for what they had been through. Moreover, they would be nested within and embraced by the emergent community of goodwill and kindness, what Buddhists call *sangha*, that seems to arise spontaneously when people practice mindfulness together. That was the vision underlying what we came to think of more and more as a *participatory medicine*, one that involved recruiting the interior resources of the patient as a vital complement to whatever medical or surgical treatments they were also receiving.

And since the words "medicine" and "meditation" actually share the same root meaning, it didn't seem as far-fetched a juxtaposition for a medical center and a school of medicine to be offering meditation to their patients as some might imagine, even back in 1979 when MBSR began.

Both "medicine" and "meditation" come from the Latin *mederi*, which means to cure. However, the deep Indo-European root of *mederi* carries the core meaning of to measure. This is not our usual notion of measure as an accounting of the quantitative relationship to an established standard for a particular property such as length, volume, or area. Rather, it refers to the Platonic notion that all things have their own right inward measure, the properties or "isness" that makes the object what it is. Medicine can be understood as that which restores right inward measure when it is disturbed, and meditation as the direct perception of right inward measure and the deep experiential knowing of its nature.

Hospitals are not the only dukkha magnets in our society, only the most obvious. Prisons are also dukkha magnets, the destination of too many lives shaped by dukkha and thus primed for perpetrating continual and untold suffering on others and on themselves. Happily, mindfulness programs are increasingly being offered in prisons.*

Then again, many of our institutions, such as schools and work sites, produce or attract their own particular brands of dukkha, and mindfulness-based programs of one kind or another are, of necessity, being brought into those domains with increasing frequency and quality as well. When it comes right down to it, dukkha is, as the Buddha taught, ubiquitous—a fact of life. It is *not* that "life is suffering," a widespread misinterpretation of the First Noble Truth (see the following chapter). It is that "there is the actuality of suffering" and it needs to be recognized and taken into account in order to be free from it. The only way out, as Helen Keller wisely observed, is through. The only way through is by recognizing dukkha when it appears and coming to know its nature intimately, moment by moment.

---

* See for example: Samuelson, M., Carmody, J., Kabat-Zinn, J., and Bratt, M.A. "Mindfulness-Based Stress Reduction in Massachusetts Correctional Facilities." *The Prison Journal* (2007) 87: 254–268.

Dharma

The quality of our relationship to experience and the multiple landscapes, both inner and outer, within which it unfolds starts, obviously, with ourselves.

For example, if we have a desire for the world to be more peaceful, can we take a good look and see if we can be at all peaceful ourselves? Are we prepared to notice how much of the time we may not be so peaceful and what that is all about? Can we notice how bellicose we can be at times, how belligerent, how self-centered and self-serving in the microcosm of our own life and mind? If we desire others to see more clearly, can we start by paying attention to how we see things ourselves, and whether we can actually perceive, apprehend, and understand what is happening in any moment without pre-judging or prejudice? And are we willing to admit to ourselves how difficult that can be, as well as how important?

If we wish to know something of who we are, in the spirit of Socrates's injunction to "know thyself" and Yeats's assertion that we don't, there is no way around the need to look deeply into ourselves. If we wish to change the world, perhaps we might do well to tackle change in ourselves alongside change in the world, even and especially in the face of our own resistance and reluctance and blindness to change, even and especially as we are being confronted with the law of impermanence and the inevitability of change, conditions we are subject to as individuals regardless of how much we resist or protest or try to control outcomes. If we wish to make a quantum leap to greater awareness, there is no getting around the need for us to be willing to wake up, and to care deeply about waking up.

In the same vein, if we wish for greater wisdom and kindness in the world, perhaps we could start by learning to inhabit our own body a bit more with some degree of kindness and wisdom, even for one moment just accepting ourselves as we are with kindness and compassion rather than forcing ourselves to conform to some impossible ideal. The world would immediately be different. If we wish to make a true difference in this world, perhaps we must first learn how to stand in relationship to our own lives and our own knowing, or at least learn along the way, which always amounts to the same thing, since the world does not wait for us but is unfolding along with us in intimate reciprocity. And if we wish to grow or change or heal in any way, perhaps to be less strident or acquisitive, or more confident or generous, perhaps we must first taste silence and stillness, and know that drinking deeply at their wells is itself healing and transformative through embracing in awareness itself whatever we find *here* in this moment, including our most deeply ingrained and unconscious tendencies.

All of this has been known for centuries. But liberative practices such as meditation were for the most part sequestered for all those centuries in monasteries under the stewardship of diverse cultural and religious traditions. For various reasons, including the vast distances lying between them geographically and culturally, and because of the distance between themselves as renunciates of the secular world and that world, these monasteries tended to be isolated, sometimes secretive about their practices, and perhaps in some cases parochial and exclusive rather than universal. At least until now.

Now, in this era, everything that has ever been discovered by human beings is out there for our investigation as it has never been before. In particular, Buddhist meditation and its associated wisdom tradition, known variously as Buddhadharma, or simply the Dharma, is available to us now as never before, and is touching the lives of millions of Americans and other Westerners in ways that would have been unimaginable forty or fifty years ago.

What the Buddhists call the Dharma is an ancient force in this world, much like the Gospels, except that it has nothing to do in essence with religious conversion or with organized religion for that matter, or even with Buddhism per se, if one wants to think of Buddhism as a religion at all. But like the Gospels, it is literally good news.

The very word "dharma," which means variously the teachings of the Buddha, the lawfulness of the universe, and "the way things are," has found its way into our language in the past century through Jack Kerouac's famous characterization of himself and his beat friends as "Dharma Bums," through the poet Allen Ginsberg's appellation of Dharma Lion, and through the marketing of it for a time as a novel woman's name in a television show, displayed prominently in subway stations and on the side of buses, as happens so often in America.

The dharma was originally articulated by the Buddha in what he referred to as the Four Noble Truths. He elaborated on this foundational teaching throughout his lifetime. It continues to be passed down and elaborated on to this day in unbroken lineages and streams within all the various Buddhist traditions. In some ways it is appropriate to characterize dharma as resembling scientific knowledge, ever growing, ever changing, yet with a core body of methods, observations, and natural laws distilled from thousands of years of inner exploration through highly disciplined self-observation and self-inquiry, a careful and precise recording and mapping of experiences encountered in investigating the nature of the mind, and direct empirical testing and confirming of the results.

However, the lawfulness of the dharma is such that, in order for it to be dharma, it cannot be exclusively Buddhist, any more than the law of gravity is English because of Newton or Italian because of Galileo, or the laws of thermodynamics Austrian because of Boltzmann. The contributions of these and other scientists who discovered and described natural laws always transcend their particular cultures because they concern nature pure and simple, and nature is one seamless and ultimately deeply mysterious whole, a wholeness that we ourselves are not outside of, but rather very much nested within.

The Buddha's elaboration of the lawfulness of the dharma transcends his particular time and culture of origin in the same way, even though a religion grew out of it, albeit a peculiar one from the Western point of view, as it is not based on worshiping a supreme deity. Mindfulness and dharma are best thought of as universal descriptions of the functioning of the human mind and heart regarding the quality of one's attention in relationship to the experience of suffering and the potential for well-being (*eudaemonia*) and wisdom. They apply equally wherever there are human minds, just as the laws of physics apply equally everywhere in our universe (as far as we know), or Noam Chomsky's universal generative grammar is applicable across all languages in the elaboration of human speech.

And from the point of view of its universality, it is helpful to recall that the Buddha himself was not a Buddhist. He was a healer and a revolutionary, albeit a quiet and inward one. He diagnosed our collective human dis-ease and prescribed a benevolent medicine for sanity and well-being. Given this, one might say that in order for Buddhism to be maximally effective as a dharma vehicle at this stage in the evolution of the planet and for its sorely needed medicine to be maximally effective, it may have to give up being Buddhism in any formal religious sense, or at least, give up any attachment to it in name or form. Since dharma is ultimately about non-duality, distinctions between Buddhadharma and universal dharma, or between Buddhists and non-Buddhists, cannot be fundamental. From this perspective, the particular traditions and forms in which it manifests are alive and vibrant, multiple, and continually evolving; at the same time, the essence remains, as always, formless, limitless, and one without distinction.

In fact, even the word "Buddhism" is not Buddhist in origin.

Apparently it was coined by European ethnologists, philologists, and religious scholars in the seventeenth and eighteenth centuries who were trying to fathom from the outside, through their own religious and cultural lenses and tacit assumptions, an exotic world that was largely opaque to them. For more than two thousand years, those who practiced the teachings of the Buddha, in whatever lineage, and there were many lineages, even within individual countries, all holding somewhat different interpretations of the original teachings, apparently simply referred to themselves as "followers of the Way" or "followers of the Dharma." They did not describe themselves as "Buddhists."

Coming back to Dharma as the teachings of the Buddha, the first of the Four Noble Truths he articulated after his intensive inquiry into the nature of mind was the universal prevalence of dukkha, the fundamental dis-ease of the human condition. The second was the cause of dukkha, which the Buddha attributed directly to attachment, clinging, and unexamined desire. The third was the assertion, based on his experience as the experimenter in the laboratory of his own meditation practice, that cessation of dukkha is possible, in other words, that it is possible to be completely cured of the dis-ease caused by craving, attachment, and clinging. And the fourth Noble Truth outlines a systematic approach, known as the Noble Eightfold Path, to the cessation of dukkha, the dispelling of ignorance, and, thus, to liberation. The four taken together actually reflect an ancient medical perspective that is still very much in use today: *diagnosis* (first Noble Truth); *etiology* (second Noble Truth); *prognosis* (third Noble Truth); and *treatment plan* (fourth Noble Truth). The prognosis is stated as very positive, namely that liberation from suffering and greed, hatred, and delusion is possible. And the treatment plan outlines the recommended approach.

Mindfulness is one of the eight practice elements of the Eightfold Path, the one unifying and informing all the others. All together, the eight practices are wise or "right" view, wise thinking, wise speech, wise action, wise livelihood, wise effort, wise mindfulness, and wise concentration. Each contains all the others. They are different aspects of one seamless whole. Thich Nhat Hanh puts it this way:

> When Right Mindfulness is present, the Four Noble Truths and the seven other elements of the Eightfold Path are also present.

THICH NHAT HANH

THE STRESS REDUCTION CLINIC
AND MBSR

Harking back to dukkha and dis-ease, if I hadn't known it before simply from my own meditation practice and observing my own incessant tendencies to go unconscious and be caught up and completely entangled in the turbulence of the thinking mind and reactive emotions, working in a stress reduction clinic soon confirmed how widespread the dis-ease of unawareness really is, and how hungry we are to set it right, how starved we are for a consistent, authentic, wholehearted experiencing of being alive, of being undivided, how starved we are for peace of mind, and how desirous of finding some relief from what often seems like a treadmill of endless physical and emotional pain.

All these and countless other faces of dukkha would arise in conversation with people who came for intake interviews before joining the program. I would merely ask as an opener, "What brings you to Stress Reduction?" and then keep quiet and listen. If the person feels met, seen, and accepted as he or she is, such a question invites speaking from the heart. It carries the felt recognition and acknowledgment that there may be limitless depths to one's suffering—or at least, that it can feel that way.

I learned from this listening that our patients came to the Stress Reduction Clinic for a lot of different reasons that, in the end, were really just one reason: to be whole again, to recapture a spark they once felt they had, or felt they never had but always wanted. They came because they wanted to learn how to relax, how to relieve some of their stress, how to lessen physical pain or learn to live better with it; how to find peace of mind and recover a sense of well-being.

They came because they wanted to take charge in their own lives and get off their pain medication or their anti-anxiety medication, and not be, as they often said, "so nervous and uptight." People came to the clinic because they had been diagnosed with heart disease, or cancer, or chronic pain conditions, or a host of other medical problems that were having an untoward influence on their lives and their freedom to pursue their dreams. They came because they were finally open, often out of desperation, to doing something about it for themselves, something that no one else on the planet could do for them, including their doctors, namely, take charge in their lives and do what they could on their own as a vital complement to what traditional allopathic medicine was able to offer, in the hope of getting stronger, healthier, somehow perhaps also wiser, inwardly and outwardly.

They came because aspects of their lives or their bodies or both weren't working for them anymore and because they knew that medicine could only do so much for them and that it wasn't going to be enough, had not been enough up to now. They came because their doctors conferred a legitimacy on squarely naming and facing up to the stress and pain in their lives and doing something about it simply by referring them to us. They came because our clinic was right there in the hospital and therefore mindfulness and stress reduction, meditation, yoga, and all the interior work they would be invited to engage in, much of it in silence, could be seen as an integral part of mainstream medicine and health care and thus, as legitimate approaches for dealing with their problems.

And perhaps above all, they came, and stayed, because we somehow managed to create an atmosphere in the room that invited a deep and openhearted listening, an atmosphere that the participants could recognize immediately as benign, empathic, respectful, and accepting. That kind of feeling tone, unfortunately, can be an all-too-rare experience in a busy medical center.

Because we gave everybody plenty of time to respond to that one question, "What brings you here?" most were willing, even happy to speak honestly and openly, often with great poignancy, of their malaise and dis-ease, of feeling lost or overwhelmed, victimized or in some way lacking, far beyond the cancer diagnosis or pain condition or heart problem listed as the primary diagnosis and reason for the referral. Their stories frequently revealed the poignant suffering of the heart that accompanies not being seen or honored by others in childhood, and of coming to adulthood without feeling their own goodness or beauty or worthiness. And of course, they spoke movingly of the suffering of the body...from chronic back pain, neck pain, face pain, leg pain, many different forms of cancer, HIV and AIDS, heart disease, and a myriad of somatic maladies, compounded in many cases by the suffering of the mind from chronic anxiety and panic, from depression and disappointment, from grief, confusion, exhaustion, chronic irritability and tension, and a host of sometimes overwhelmingly afflictive emotional states.

The good news, as people going through the MBSR program have discovered for themselves time and again over the years, and as documented in an ever-increasing number of medical studies, not just from our own clinic but from mindfulness-based programs in hospitals and clinics around the world, is that each and every one of us can have a hand, finally, in facing and embracing the fullness of what we are as human beings, in affirming that whoever we are, it is possible to wake up to what is hidden and opaque, frightened and frightening in us that shapes our lives whether we know it or not, and to awaken as well to other, healthier, saner longings that call to us from the depths of our own hearts and let them flower in our lives in ways that are restorative and healing, and in many cases, dramatically symptom reducing. My colleagues and I in MBSR clinics around the country and around the world have seen this happen for countless people suffering with unthinkable levels of stress, pain, illness, and unimaginable life circumstances and histories, from "the full catastrophe," the full-spectrum poignancy of the human condition itself in all its rending and unendingly complex urgency and specificity.

Whether big or little, gross or subtle, the degree of transformation that can take place in people over a relatively short time never ceases to astonish me. I can sometimes see it unfolding in myself as well when my senses don't take leave of me or I of them. And amazingly, at times I can even manage to catch the taking leave when it does occur and thereby restore a measure of momentary or even sustained balance and clarity.

Embracing the full catastrophe of the human condition and facing what is perhaps most unwanted but nevertheless already present once it has occurred is part of waking up to our lives and to living the lives that are actually ours to live. In part, it involves refusing to let the dis-ease and the dukkha, however gross or however subtle, go unnoticed and unnamed. It involves being willing to turn toward and work with whatever arises in our experience, knowing or having faith that it is workable, especially if we are willing to do a certain kind of work ourselves, the work of awareness, which involves easing ourselves over and over again back into the present moment and all it has to offer when we learn, and when we remember, to rest in that awareness and draw upon its remarkable energies in the unfolding of our very lives, just as they are, just as we find them.

A.D.D. NATION

One manifestation of dukkha and dis-ease, increasingly prevalent in this era, is attention deficit disorder, A.D.D. for short. A.D.D. is a serious dis-regulation in the process of attention itself. It occurs in both children and adults. Forty years ago, no one had ever heard of attention deficit. In fact, such a diagnosis didn't exist. Now, it appears to be a widespread and growing affliction.

Since meditation has everything to do with the cultivation of our capacity to pay attention, you might think that the meditative perspective could shed light on possible ways to prevent or treat this condition, and indeed, that is the case. But it might also be worth stating that, from the perspective of the meditative traditions, the entire society suffers from attention deficit disorder—big time—and from its most prevalent variant, attention deficit *hyperactivity* disorder, A.D.H.D. And it is getting worse by the day. Learning how to refine our ability to pay attention and to sustain attention may no longer be a luxury but a lifeline back to what is most meaningful in our lives, what is most easily missed, ignored, denied, or run through so quickly that it could not possibly be noticed.

I have a sense that as Americans, we also tend to suffer from attention deficit in another, more subtle and subterranean way due to the particular direction our culture has taken in the past half century. That is, we are lacking and feel bereft of true caring attention from others. We are prone to feeling more and more lonely and invisible in this celebrity-obsessed entertainment culture that can be so isolating in its insularity—think of watching the fare of sitcoms and reality TV night after night, emoting off other people's lives or fantasies, or finding one's most intimate relationships online in chat rooms, or on Facebook, Snapchat, or Instagram, constantly looking for likes and approval and connection. Are we not also obsessively preoccupied with consuming—think of the incessant drive to fill up your time, to get somewhere else, or obtain what you feel you are lacking so you can feel satisfied and happy?

In our loneliness and isolation and seemingly perpetual impulse toward self-distraction in the service of finding a moment of meaningful connection, there is a deep longing, a yearning, usually unconscious or ignored, to belong, to be part of a larger whole, to not be anonymous, to be seen and known. For relationality, exchange, give-and-take, especially on an emotional plane, is how we are reminded that we have a place in this world, how we know in our hearts that we actually do belong and make a difference. It is deeply satisfying to experience meaningful connection with others. We hunger for that feeling of belonging, for the feeling that we are connected to something larger than ourselves. We hunger to be perceived by others, to be both noticed and valued for who we actually are, and not merely for what we do. And mostly we are not.

Rarely are we touched by the benevolent seeing and knowing of who we are by other people, who, for the most part, are moving too fast and are too self-preoccupied to pay attention to anyone else for long. Our way of life across suburban and rural communities tends to be insular and isolating. Even urban neighborhood culture tends to be isolating, lonely, and insecure nowadays. Children watch hour upon hour of television or disappear into computer games or smartphones rather than play in neighborhoods, in part simply to insure their safety, in part out of habit, addiction, and boredom. Their attention while tuned in to devices is an entirely passive, asocial attention, a perpetual distraction from their own interiority, and from embodied relationality. Many studies are showing that active social engagement is on the decline in children. And as adults, we may no longer know our neighbors, and we certainly don't depend on them as earlier generations did. It is the rare neighborhood that is a true community nowadays.

Even in families, in this era many parents of young children are often so stressed, so preoccupied, and so infernally busy that they are at high risk for not being present for their children, even when they are physically present. Parents are so chronically overwhelmed and distracted that they may not even see their children clearly in many moments, or even think to pick up and hold the little ones when they are distressed. So no one in the family may be consistently getting the amount of attention they need and deserve.

On the medical front, just getting your doctor to pay attention to you can be challenging, or nigh impossible in this era. Doctors have so little time for their patients. They are squeezed and stressed by their own scheduling pressures. Unintended disregard can become an occupational hazard, and an endemic condition. Good doctors guard against it knowingly as best they can, but even the best doctors are being crushed under the time pressures of medicine in this era of "managed" (read rationed and increasingly profit-driven) care.

Attention deficit was probably not so prevalent when we were hunters and gatherers for most of the 100,000-plus years of *Homo sapiens sapiens'* sojourn on Earth, or when we turned to agriculture and animal husbandry, raising grains and livestock ten thousand years ago. Note that the word *"sapiens"* itself is the present participle— indicating unfolding in the present moment—of the Latin verb *sapere*, to know, to taste, to perceive, to be wise. We are the knowing knowing species. We are the species that has the capacity to know and to know that we know, in other words, to be wise, to have a meta perspective, to be aware of being aware—or so we named ourselves, tellingly.

As noted earlier, our hunter-and-gatherer ancestors needed to pay attention constantly or they would either have starved or been eaten, gotten lost, or wound up exposed to the elements without shelter. And since the community one was born into was all there was, that capacity to pay careful attention and read the signs of the natural world was bound to include reading each other's faces, moods, and intentions. For all these reasons, any deficit in attention would have been strongly selected against in evolution. You would never have lived long enough to have children and pass on your genes.

By the same token, farmers are naturally entrained into the rhythms of the earth and of new life and the hourly need for its tending. Paying attention and attunement to these cycles of nature, of the day and of the hours and of the seasons, long before there were clocks and calendars to mark the passage of time, were critical to survival.

No wonder when we seek calmness, so many of us find it in nature. The natural world has no artifice. The tree outside the window, and the birds in it, stand only in the now, remnants of what was once pristine wilderness, which was and is, where it is still protected, timeless on the scale of the human. The natural world always defines now. We instinctively feel a part of nature because our forebears were born of it and into it, and the natural world was the only world, all there was. It offered a multiplicity of experiential dimensions for its inhabitants, all of which needed to be understood to survive, including what they sometimes called the spirit world, or the world of the gods, worlds that could be sensed even though they were usually invisible.

Changing seasons, wind and weather, light and night, mountains, rivers, trees, oceans and ocean currents, fields, plants and animals, wilderness and the wild speak to us even now. They invite us and carry us back into the present that they define and are always in (and we too, except that we forget). They help us to focus and to attend to what is important, remind us, in Mary Oliver's elegantly turned phrase, of "our place in the family of things."

But much has changed for us in the last hundred years, as we have drifted away from intimacy with the natural world and a lifetime connectedness to the community into which we were born. And that change has become even more striking in the past twenty-five or so years, with the advent and virtually (pun intended) universal adoption of the digital revolution. All our "time-saving" and enhanced connectivity devices orient us in the direction of greater speed, greater abstraction, greater dis-embodiment, greater distance, and if we are not careful, greater disconnect.

It is now harder to pay attention to any one thing and there is more to pay attention to. We are easily diverted and more easily distracted. We are continuously bombarded with texts, push notifications, appeals, deadlines, communications, and way too much information that we don't need and can't possibly take in and process. Things come at us fast and furious, relentlessly. And almost all of it is man-made; it has thought behind it, and more often than not, an appeal to either our greed or our fears. These assaults on our nervous system continually stimulate and foster desire and agitation rather than contentedness and calmness. They foster reaction rather than communion, discord rather than accord or concord, acquisitiveness rather than feeling whole and complete as we are. And above all, if we are not careful, they rob us of time, of our moments. We are continually being squeezed for time and catapulted into the future as our present moments are assaulted and consumed in the fires of endless urgency, even if it is just the urgency to get one more thing done. It can seem like there is never enough time.

In the face of all this speed and greed and somatic insensitivity, we are entrained into being more and more in our heads, trying to figure things out and stay on top of things rather than sensing how they really are. In a world that is no longer primarily natural or alive, we find ourselves continually interfacing with machines that extend our reach even as we succumb to disembodying ourselves through their addictive use, whether it is the radio in the car, the car itself, the television in the bedroom, the computer in the office and increasingly in the kitchen, and the smart phone everywhere.

The relentless acceleration of our way of life over the past few generations has made focusing in on anything at all something of a lost art. That loss has been compounded by the digital revolution, which—think back just a few short years, if you are old enough—rapidly found its way into our everyday lives in the form of home computers, fax machines, beepers, cell phones, cell phones with cameras, palm devices for personal organization, laptops, 24/7 high-speed connectivity, the Internet and its World Wide Web, and of course, e-mail, all now increasingly wireless, not that long ago an unthinkable dream, the stuff of science fiction. For all the undeniable convenience, usefulness, access, efficiency, improved coordinating, information, organization, entertainment, and ease of online shopping, banking, and communication these digital developments bring with them, this colossal technological revolution that has barely even begun has already irreversibly transfigured how we live our lives, whether we realize it or not.

And there is no question that it has barely begun. Yet already it has thoroughly transformed the home and the way we work—many people now sit in front of consoles, stare at screens, and type and click on icons all day long, and day after day; to a first approximation, that is what most work has turned into for a huge segment of the workforce—and has upped the ante in terms of how much work we can get done in a day and therefore our expectations for the attainment of goals and for the immediate delivery of whatever it is we, or "they," want. This new way of working and living has inundated us all of a sudden with endless options, endless opportunities for interruption, distraction, highly enabled "response ability" (every pun intended), and a kind of free-floating urgency attached to even the most trivial of events. The to-do list grows ever longer, and we are always rushing through this moment to get to the next.

All this threatens to erode our ability and inclination to sustain attention and thereby to know things in a deep way *before* initiating some kind of action. We see this lack of attention when, on e-mail, we click *send*, only in the next second to remember that we forgot to attach what we just said we would, or decide we didn't really want to say what we just did, or that we really wanted to say something we didn't...but it is already gone.

The technology itself undermines any time we might be inclined to take for reflection. It fosters a sometimes irresistible urge to get it out and scroll down to the next thing, move on to the next item in our in-box. We might sigh inwardly and then let it be, or send a correction if possible. What else can we do with prematurely escaped e-mails?

But in this way, a pervasive mediocrity can creep into our everyday discourse and interactions, especially if we are not mindful of these insidious choices we are making from one moment to the next. For we are literally, as some A.D.D. specialists have observed, being driven to distraction by all our delicious opportunities and choices. We even interrupt ourselves, often moment by moment, in our compulsive multitasking, so foreign has our capacity and desire to concentrate the mind and direct it toward one object become.

We drive ourselves to distraction and the human world drives us to distraction in ways the natural world in which we grew up as a species never did. The human world, for all its wonders and profound gifts, also bombards us with more and more useless things to entice us, seduce us, pique our fancy, appeal to our endless desire for becoming. It erodes the chances of us being satisfied with being in any moment, with actually appreciating this moment without having to fill it with anything or move on to the next one. It robs us of time even as we complain we don't have any. It has given rise to a dance of inattention and instability of mind. Oh, that we could work at being undistracted—and be undistracted when we work.

It is telling and actually tragic that large numbers of young children are now being medicated for A.D.D. and A.D.H.D., down to even three year olds. Could it be that in many of these cases, it is the adults who are entraining the children into distraction and hyperactivity, if such behaviors are not actually normative for these times, and therefore strictly speaking, normal under the circumstances? Maybe the children's behavior is only a symptom of a much more pervasive dis-ease of family life, and life in general in this era, as is likely the case for the rampant obesity epidemic we are seeing in children and adults.

If parents are rarely present because we are so busy and overwhelmed, and if we are lost in our heads even when we are physically present, and if we are away at work most of the time, including evenings and weekends, or on the phone a lot when we are home, and also juggling all the physical and organizational needs of the household, perhaps our children, even the very little ones, are suffering from outright parent deprivation and a huge, almost genetic grief behind it. Perhaps there is a deficit of parental attention, a deficit of actual living, breathing, feeling, body-snuggling, reliable rather than erratic, undistracted presence.

After all, it is the big people's universe, or so we big people tend to think. So if we adults are impelled to be distracted constantly to one degree or another, and have a hard time focusing on any one thing for long, is it any wonder that more and more children might be that way too since their rhythms from the time they are born are, to an extraordinary degree, especially as newborns and infants, so attuned to ours?

Or perhaps, in some cases, the children are not really suffering from A.D.D. at all, at least before they get phones and instant messaging. They may be just normal children with a lot of energy, as some temperaments exhibit. But they may now be perceived, even diagnosed as classroom problems, behavioral deviants with A.D.D. or A.D.H.D. because the adults no longer have the time or inclination or patience to deal consistently with the normal exuberance and challenges of childhood.

So many of us feel trapped by our circumstances, yet at the same time also addicted to the speed at which our lives are unfolding. Even our stress and distress can feel oddly satisfying or outright intoxicating. So we may be reluctant to slow down and give ourselves over to the present moment, to attend fully to our children's needs when they are in conflict with our own, even though our children's needs are very real and ever changing, not because they have a behavioral disorder, but because they are children.

If anything, our children may be succumbing to a dis-ease acquired from having to live with us in our A.D.D./A.D.H.D. households and having to go to overly regimented A.D.D./A.D.H.D. schools with disembodied curricula, dominated by huge amounts of mostly fragmented, unintegrated information. And then, as a product of this initiation, they are supposed to be equipped to find their way into our A.D.D./A.D.H.D. society and connect in meaningful ways to work and relationships and their own lives. Even if this is only a partially accurate characterization, it might give anybody a headache, if not panic attacks, just thinking about it.

24/7 Connectivity

With the tiniest bit of attention, it is easy to realize that our world is changing radically right under our very noses in ways that have never before been experienced by the human nervous system. In light of the enormity of these changes and their impact on our lives and families and work, it might be a good idea to reflect from time to time on just how they may be affecting our lives. For that matter, it might be a good idea to bring mindfulness to the whole domain of 24/7 connectivity and what it is doing for us and to us.

My guess is that, for the most part, we have hardly been noticing. We have been too caught up in adapting to the new possibilities and challenges, learning to use the new technologies to get more done and get it done faster and perhaps even better, and in the process, becoming completely dependent on them, even addicted. And whether we realize it or not, we are being swept along in a current of time acceleration that shows no signs of slowing down. The technology, so touted to produce gains in efficiency and leisure, threatens to rob us of both if it hasn't already done so. Who do you know who has more leisure? The very concept seems foreign to our time, a throwback to the 1950s.

It is said that the pace of our lives now is being driven by an inexorable exponential acceleration known as Moore's law (after Intel founder Gordon Moore, who first stated it) governing the size and speed of integrated circuits. Every eighteen months, the computing power and speed of the next generation of microprocessors increases by a factor of two while their size decreases by a factor of two and their cost remains about the same. Think of it: increasing processing speed, greater and greater miniaturization, and cheaper and cheaper electronics, with no end in sight. This combination proffers a seduction in computer systems for work and home, consumer products, games, and portable electronic devices that can easily lead to outright addiction and the loss of all sense of measure and direction as we respond willy-nilly to the increasing volumes of e-mail, voice mail, faxes, pages, and cell phone traffic coming in from all corners of the planet. True, aside from the mountains of junk and aggressive ads and the bombardment of our senses virtually everywhere so there is no escape, much of what comes to us is from people we care about and with whom we want to stay connected. But what about balance, and how do we regulate the pace of instant and ubiquitous connectivity, and the expectations of instantaneous responding?

With digital devices and smart phones, we are now able to be so connected that we can be in touch with anyone and everyone at any time, do business anywhere, get texts and calls, or check e-mail anywhere and at any time. But has it ever crossed your mind that in the process, we run the risk of never being in touch with ourselves? In the overall seduction, we can easily forget that our primary connection to life is through our own interiority—the experiencing of our own body and all our senses, including the mind, which allow us to touch and be touched by the world, and to act appropriately in response to it. And for that, we need moments that are not filled with anything, in which we do not jump to get in one more phone call or send one more e-mail, or plan one more event, or add to our to-do list, even if we can. Moments of reflection, of mulling, of thinking things over, of thoughtfulness.

Within the urgency and tyranny of connectivity, what about connectivity to ourselves? Are we becoming so connected to everybody else that we are never where we actually are? We are at the beach on the cell phone, so are we there? We are walking down the street on the cell phone, so are we there? We are driving on the cell phone, so are we there? Do we have to let the possibility of being in our life go out the window in the face of the speedup in our pace of life and the possibilities for instant and endless connection?

What about *not* connecting with anyone in our "in-between" moments? What about realizing that there are actually no in-between moments at all? What about being in touch with who is on *this* end of the call, not the other end? What about calling ourselves up for a change, and checking in, seeing what we are up to? We don't even need our phone for that, although increasingly, there are mindfulness apps to remind us to drop in. But while those might be useful for developing or deepening a formal meditation practice, including the ones that I developed specifically to accompany this book (see page 195), what about just being in touch with how *we* are feeling in any and every moment, even in those moments when we may be feeling numb, or overwhelmed, or bored, or disjointed, or anxious or depressed, or needing to get one more thing done?

What about being connected to our bodies, and to the universe of sensations through which we sense and know the outer landscape? What about lingering for more than the most mindless and automatic of moments with awareness of whatever is arising in any particular moment in the mind: our emotions and moods, our feelings, our thoughts, our beliefs? What about lingering not just with their content, but also with their feeling tone, their actuality as energies and significant events in our lives, as huge reservoirs of information for self-understanding, huge opportunities for catalyzing transformation, for living authentically in accordance with what we are experiencing moment by moment, and with what we know and understand? What about cultivating a bigger picture that includes ourselves on any and every level, even if the picture is always a work in progress, always tentative, always changing, always emerging or failing to emerge, sometimes with clarity, sometimes not?

Much of the time, our newfound technological connectivity

serves no real purpose, just habit, and pushes the bounds of absurdity, as in the *New Yorker* cartoon:

> A train station at rush hour. People pouring out of the train and people pouring onto the train. All with cell phones to their ears. The caption: "I'm getting on the train now" "I'm getting off the train now."

Who are these people? (Oh yes, I almost forgot, it's all of us.) What is wrong with just getting on the train or getting off the train, without that vital piece of information being communicated? Doesn't anyone just get off a plane now and meet their party the old-fashioned way and just have the cell phone for back-up? From my casual observations once the plane lands, the answer is no. Pretty soon, if we're not careful, it will be, "I'm in the bathroom now. I'm washing my hands now." Do we really need to know?

If we were telling *ourselves*, it might just be a mindful noting of our experience, and therefore quite useful in cultivating awareness of embodied experience unfolding in the present moment. I am getting on the train (and knowing it). I am getting off the train (and knowing it). I am going to the bathroom (and knowing it). I am feeling the water on my hands (and knowing it). I am appreciating where clean water comes from and how precious it is. That is embodied wakefulness. With practice, we may come to see that the personal pronoun is not so necessary. It is just getting on, getting off, going, feeling, knowing, knowing, knowing....

Tell someone else? Who needs it? It can annihilate the moment through distraction, diversion, and reification. Somehow, being alone in and with our experience is no longer deemed sufficient, even though it is our life in that moment.

It does give one pause...maybe just the pause we need to realize our essential but so easily missed connectedness with the body, the breath, with the unadulterated, analog, non-digitized world of nature, with this moment as it is and with who we actually are.

This is not to say that much of the technology we are immersed in nowadays is not amazing and extremely useful. Cell phones allow parents to stay in touch with their children wherever they are, day or night. They alerted passengers on one highjacked plane on 9/11 to what their situation was, and apparently led passengers on the fourth plane to prevent it from hitting its target. Cell phones allow us to find each other and to coordinate our activities in amazing and useful ways. But they are also a major cause of car accidents, as people are now more preoccupied with their phone conversations (and, according to a recent study, even more so with fiddling with the radio dial, with eating, and with grooming themselves) than they are with driving safely, or even knowing where they are as they are driving. It adds a whole new level of meaning to being out to lunch...dangerously so, bordering on the criminal in many cases. (Phone to ear: "Oops! Sorry. I just almost ran you over. I didn't see you crossing in front of me. I was in the middle of a heavy conversation with my accountant, my lawyer, my mother, my business partner.") And that is to say nothing about the huge issues of privacy digital technology is confronting us with, that our every purchase and movement can be tracked and analyzed and our personal habits profiled and catalogued in ways that we can scarcely imagine, and that may redefine entirely what we consider to be the realm of the private. At the very least, it means receiving more and more catalogues in the mail.

Computers and printers and their amazing software capabilities, coupled with the capacity to exchange documents instantly by e-mail anywhere and everywhere and access information instantly that before might have taken days to get at our very fingertips, in many cases allow us individually and collectively to get more work done in a day than we might have gotten done in a week or even a month twenty-five years ago, and perhaps better work too. I am not by any stretch of the imagination advocating a Luddite-like condemnation of technological development and romantically wishing to turn the clock back to a simpler age. But I do think it is important for us to be mindful of all the new and increasingly powerful ways available to us, with more on the way every day and every year, through which we can and will be able to lose ourselves in the addictive pull of the outer and forget about the inner, thereby becoming even more out of touch with ourselves.

The more we are entrained into the outer world in all these new and increasingly rapid ways that our nervous system has never before encountered, the more important it may be for us to develop a robust counterbalance of the inner world, one that calms and tunes the nervous system and puts it in the service of living wisely, both for ourselves and for others. This counterbalance can be cultivated by bringing greater mindfulness to the body, to the mind, and to our experiences at the interface between outer and inner, including the very moments in which we are using the technology to stay connected, or in which the impulse to do so is arising. Otherwise, we may wind up at very high risk of living robotic lives, where we no longer even have time to contemplate who is doing all this doing, who is getting somewhere more desirable, and is it really?

CONTINUAL PARTIAL ATTENTION

Linda Stone, a former Microsoft researcher, was quoted by Thomas Friedman in the *New York Times* describing our present state of mind as one of "continual partial attention." Friedman himself gets personal: "I love that phrase. It means that while you are answering your e-mail and talking to your kid, your cell phone rings and you have a conversation. Now you are involved in a continuous flow of interactions in which you can only partially concentrate on each."

"If being fulfilled is about committing yourself to someone else, or some experience, that requires a level of sustained attention," said Ms. Stone. And that is what we are losing the skills for, because we are constantly scanning the world for opportunities and we are constantly in fear of missing something better. That has become incredibly spiritually depleting.

Friedman goes on:

I am struck by how many people call my office, ask if I'm in, and, if not, immediately ask to be connected to my cell phone or pager (I carry neither). You're never out anymore. The assumption now is that you're always in. Out is over. Now you are always in. And when you are always in you are always on.

And when you are always on, what are you most like? A computer server....

The problem is that human beings simply are not designed to be like computer servers. For one thing, they are designed to sleep eight hours a night....As Jeff Garten, dean of the Yale School of Management and author of ... *The Mind of the CEO*, said, "Maybe it's not time for us to adapt or die, but for the technology to adapt or die."

But that kind of adaptation is not likely without a major commitment to becoming more mindful. Perhaps it has not escaped your notice that nowadays, more and more, in large measure due to the innovations in office technology, there is no end to work. There is no longer a workday, as work and our capacity to do it anywhere expands into all hours of the clock. There is no longer a workweek for many of us, and no boundary between the week and the weekend. There is no longer a workplace, as anyplace, airplanes, restaurants, vacation homes, hotels, walking down the street, biking along a bike path becomes a work site and a cell phone, e-mail, and Internet portal. As a full-page advertisement in the *New York Times* put it ten years ago, "When Microsoft Office goes wireless, an amazing thing happens. You can now take your workplace anywhere."

Yes. This is wonderful and convenient and unbelievably helpful in many ways, and in the past ten years or so, work has only gotten more that way. I am not criticizing it so much as suggesting that we bring awareness to how the lure of incoming and outgoing demands for our attention and input is influencing our lives, and to remember that it might be possible to make moment-to-moment choices in favor of greater balance. The more we make use of the technology, the more we come to depend on it and become entrained into its ever-accelerating lure, the more we need to ask ourselves, "When is our time for us?" When is our time for just being? For living an analog life? When is family time important enough not to be interrupted or carried away from? When is there time for just walking or biking, or eating, or shopping, and just being with what is unfolding in that moment without extraneous intrusions or the need to get the next thing done at the same time to further our never-ending agendas to accomplish, or just to fill up (we also say "kill") time when we are bored? And would we know what to do with such time any longer, how to be in it, if it appeared? Or would we reflexively pick up a newspaper or phone someone, or start clicking the remote—as we ourselves get more and more remote from real life?

A few examples from the business section of the Sunday *New York Times*, from 2004, three years before the advent of the iPhone in 2007.

"Ten years ago, you had to be in the office 12 hours," said Bruce P. Mehlman, assistant commerce secretary for technology policy and a former executive at Cisco Systems, who said he now spends 10 hours a day at work, giving him more time with his wife and three children, while also making use of his wireless laptop, BlackBerry and mobile phone.

"I get to help my kids get dressed, feed them breakfast, give them a bath and read them stories at night," he said. He can also have Lego air fights—a game in which he and his 5-year-old son have imaginary dogfights with Lego airplanes.

Both love the game, and it has an added benefit for Dad: he can play with one hand while using the other to talk on the phone or check e-mail. The multitasking maneuver occasionally requires a trick: although Mr. Mehlman usually lets his son win the Lego air battle, he sometimes allows himself to win, which forces his son to spend a few minutes putting his plane back together. "While he is rebuilding his plane, I check my e-mail on the BlackBerry," Mr. Mehlman explained.

Charles Lax, a 44-year-old venture capitalist, uses technology to keep up in a "race against time" with his well-financed competitors. By his own admission, he is "Always On." On his office desk is a land-line telephone, a mobile phone, a laptop computer connected to several printers, and a television, often tuned to CNN or CNBC. At his side is the aptly named Sidekick, a mobile device [now surpassed and made obsolete by the smart phone] that serves as camera, calendar, address book, instant-messaging gadget and fallback phone. It can browse the internet and receive e-mail. He has been known to pick it up whenever it chirps at him—and he acknowledges having used it to check e-mail in the men's room.

There is no down-time in the car, either. "I talk on the phone, but I have a headset," Mr. Lax said. Does he do anything else, like using his Sidekick to read e-mail? "I won't be quoted as saying what else I do because it could get me arrested," he said, laughing.

Mr. Lax said he loved the constant stimulation. "It's instant gratification," he said, and it staves off boredom. "I use it when I'm in a waiting situation—if I am standing in line, waiting to be served lunch, or getting takeout coffee at Starbucks. And my God, at the airport, it's disastrous to have to wait there.

"Being able to send an e-mail in real time is just—" Mr. Lax paused. "Can you hold for a second? My other line is ringing."

When he returned, he said he shared this way of working with many venture capitalists. "We all suffer a kind of A.D.D.," he said. "It's a bit of a joke, but it's true. We are easily bored. We have lots of things going on at the same time." He even checks his e-mail during workouts at the gym.

The technology gives him a way to direct his excess energy. "It is a kind of Ritalin," he said. But he said technology dependence could have its down side. "I'm in meetings all the time with people who are focused on what they're doing on their computers, not on the presentation."*

To the degree that we become addicted to the technology, seduced into the computer server mode, to at least that degree we will need to assert the primacy of our interior lives and the power of full moment-by-moment attention in connecting with ourselves and the world as it unfolds moment by moment. If we are never away from e-mail and smart phones, if we are continually seduced into mindless multitasking, then "out" may be over, as Friedman says, but "in" may be over too, rendered meaningless, as we cease knowing how to be fully present, or how to give our wholly undivided attention to one matter, or even that it might matter.

It has been shown time and time again that effective multitasking is a myth—performance on every one of the tasks in question degrades as our attention shuttles back and forth among competing demands.

So the challenge of the moment is really the question of whether we can be "in" for ourselves ever again? Can presence of mind be sustained over time? Can we pay attention to just one thing, the matter at hand, whatever it may be? Are we ever going to be off duty, so we can be rather than just do? And when might that be?

If not the whispered longing and innate wisdom of our own hearts, what and who will ever call us home to ourselves anymore?

And will we need the phone company or some embedded microchip somewhere, in the future, to do even that?

---

* See my colleague Judson Brewer's book, *The Craving Mind: From Cigarettes to Smart-Phones to Love—Why We Get Hooked & How We Can Break Bad Habits* (New Haven, CT: Yale University Press).

THE "SENSE" OF TIME PASSING

Have you ever noticed that the inward sense of time slows dramatically when you are off in some unfamiliar place engaged in some adventurous undertaking? Go to a foreign city for a week and do a lot of different things, and it seems when you get back that you've been gone for much longer. One day can seem like a whole week, and a week like a month, you did so much, and enjoyed yourself so thoroughly.

You can have a similar experience if you go off camping in the wilderness. Every experience is novel. It's not "sightseeing" but still, every sight you see is for the first time. Because of that, the frequency of notable or what we think of as "noteworthy" moments is higher than it might be at home. And of course, there are fewer of the usual household distractions, unless you brought a Winnebago and your satellite dish or laptop. Meanwhile, the people who stayed at home had a regular week more or less, and it seemed to go by for them like a flash, as if you had hardly left and now you are already back.

According to Ray Kurzweil, computer wizard, futurist, artificial intelligence proponent, and inventor of sense enhancers for the sensory-impaired, our internal, subjective sense of time passing is calibrated by the interval between what we feel or sense as "milestone" or noteworthy events, along with "the degree of chaos" in the system. He calls this the Law of Time and Chaos. When order decreases and chaos (the quantity of disordered events relative to the process) increases in a system, time (the time between salient events) slows down. And when order increases and chaos decreases in a system, time (the time between salient events) speeds up. This corollary, which he calls the Law of Accelerating Returns, describes evolutionary processes, like the evolution of species, or of technologies, or computing power.

Babies and young children have lots of milestone events happening in those formative years and the frequency of such events decreases over time, even as the level of chaos in the system (say, for example, unpredictable life events) increases. The interval between milestone events is short and thus the felt experience of childhood is one of timelessness, or of time passing very slowly. We are hardly aware of it, we are so much in the present moment. As we get older, the spaced intervals (time) between noteworthy developmental milestones seems to stretch out more and more, and the present moment often seems empty and unfulfilling, always the same. Subjectively, it feels like time is speeding up as we age because our reference frame is growing longer.

So if you wanted to slow down the inner feeling of your life passing, and perhaps passing you by, there are two ways to do it. One is to fill your life with as many novel and hopefully "milestone" experiences as you can. Many people are addicted to this path of living, always looking for the next big experience to make life worthwhile, whether it is the big trip to the exotic location, extreme sports, or just the next gourmet dinner.

The other way to slow down the felt sense of time passing is to make more of your ordinary moments notable and noteworthy by taking note of them. This also reduces the chaos and increases the order in the mind. The tiniest moments can become veritable milestones. If you were really present with and inhabiting your moments with full awareness as they were unfolding, no matter what was happening, you would discover that each moment is unique and novel and therefore, momentous. Your experience of time would slow time down.

You might even find yourself stepping out of the subjective experience of time passing altogether, as you open to the timeless quality of the present moment. Since there are an astronomically large number of moments in the rest of your life, no matter how old you are, the more you are here for them, the more vivid life becomes. The richer the moments themselves and shorter the interval between them, the slower the passage of time from the point of view of your experience of it, and the "longer" your life becomes, as you are here for more of your moments.

Now interestingly, there is yet another way in which the sense of time passing slows down. This way feels really bad. That is when we are caught up in depression, emotional turmoil, and unhappiness. If things don't go well on our vacation, a week, even a day, can seem interminable because we don't want to be here. Things are not going according to plan. Our expectations are not being fulfilled, and we are in a seemingly ceaseless struggle with the way things are because they are not as we want them to be.

Time then feels like a weight, and we can't wait—to get home, or for outer circumstances to change, for the rain to let up, whatever it is that we absolutely have to have happen in order to feel fulfilled, to feel happy. Whether away or at home, when we fall into depression and its related mood states, we may struggle to do things but everything we do seems empty and a drag on us, everything is an effort and time itself drags and drags us down, into the doldrums. It feels as if a significant, momentous, uplifting event will never happen, that there are no more developmental milestones to be achieved or experienced.

In the domain of the outer world, Kurzweil argues that our technologies are evolving at an exponential rate, following the Law of Accelerating Returns (of which Moore's Law is a case in point), and thus the milestone developments in technology are coming faster and faster. Since our lives and our society are now so intimately entwined with our machines, this acceleration in the rate of change itself is simultaneously entraining our lives into an increasingly accelerating pace, which is why things not only seem to be but actually are going faster and faster.

We are having to adapt to an ever-quickening pace of working and ever-more-demanding needs to process huge amounts of information quickly, communicate about it effectively, and get important, or at least urgent, things done. Even our options for being entertained have expanded at an ever-accelerating pace, providing us with increasing and increasingly instant choices in our attempts to find moments of relaxation, distraction, and satisfaction. And it is only getting faster as time goes on.

*

Many digital engineers believe, Kurzweil among them, that as machines are programmed to become more and more "intelligent," in the sense of capable of learning and modifying their output on the basis of their input ("experience"), machines themselves rather than people will design the next generations of machines. This is already happening in many industries. Moreover, what with the potential for silicon implants (such as memory "upgrades"), robots that simulate thinking and perhaps even feelings, nanotechnology, and genetic engineering, some prescient digital engineers are warning that evolution has gone beyond the human and now includes the evolution of machines, such that the era of human beings as we know and use the term "human" may be coming to a close, and more quickly than any of us realize or can fathom.*

If this has even a remote possibility of being true, then perhaps we had best explore the full repertoire of our humanity and our evolutionary inheritance while we still have it to explore, which would include asking questions about how valuable it is to us as a society to

---

* See for example, Tegmark, M. *Life 3.0: Being Human in the Age of Artificial Intelligence* (New York, Knopf, 2017).

consciously regulate this technological evolution so that it does not extinguish those aspects of our billion or so years of genetic inheritance, and perhaps 100,000 years as *Homo sapiens sapiens* and mere 5,000 years or so of what we call "civilization" that we consider important and valuable.

We have been extraordinarily precocious as a species, especially in our development and use of tools, language, art forms, thought, science, and technology. But in other arenas, we have yet to avail ourselves, on anything approaching a global scale, of our potential for self-knowing, for wisdom, and for compassion, for example. These dimensions of our inheritance are innate to our large brains and our extraordinary bodies, but so far, they remain woefully underdeveloped. We may have a very hard time adapting to what we are facing as a species in the coming decades unless we find ways to cultivate those aspects of our own minds, find ways to slow time down both inwardly and outwardly, and use our moments and our capacity for clear seeing and for wisdom to better advantage.

*

Coming back to the experience of time passing, mindfulness can restore our moments to us by reminding us that it is possible and even valuable to linger with them, dwell in them, feel them through all our senses and know them in awareness. That awareness, we could say, is experientially outside of time, in the eternal now, the present. As such, moments spent in silent wakefulness, without having to have anything happen next, without even any purpose other than being alive and awake enough to appreciate life as it is in this moment, afford us a critical degree of balance and clarity which is almost always being undermined by the turbulence and tenacity of our inner and outer addictions. In this way, mindfulness slows down or even stops for a time the felt sense of time passing. It can also give us new ways to hold and look deeply into what is happening in the exterior landscape and our responses to it, including our vulnerability to and our entrainment into what is unfolding in the technological, social, and political realms. And in the interior landscape, mindfulness gives us a chance to see beyond the emotional reactions and patterns that afflict us with misery and a sense of despair and loneliness. It offers us new opportunities for working with the mystery of both the emptiness and the fullness of time, and time passing.

*

"People say life is too short when it's actually too long. These places [coffeeshops, stores] prove it. They exist solely to drain off excess time."

So why is Mr. Seinfeld doing this [struggling to develop a stand-up comedy routine] to himself? Why doesn't he just take his mega-millions and go to St. Bart's for a few years?

"I do think about that a lot. The reason is, I guess, is that I really do love it. I love doing stand-up. It's fun and it uses everything you have as a human being. And it all happens right here and now. The degree to which you achieve anything is immediately reflected right back to you in that moment."

JERRY SEINFELD, IN THE *NEW YORK TIMES*
MAGAZINE

AWARENESS HAS NO CENTER AND
NO PERIPHERY

It is hard to notice but also hard not to notice that awareness, when we dwell within it, has no center and no periphery. In that way, it resembles space itself and what we know of the boundaryless structure of the universe.

Yet, despite Galileo, the Copernican revolution, and Hubble's astounding discovery of the expansion of the universe in all directions from every location, we still tend to think and feel and speak as if the cosmos were centered on our little planet. We speak of the sun rising in the east and setting in the west, and that convention works very well for us in getting us through the day, even though we know full well that that is not what is actually happening at all, and that actually the planet is rotating us into and out of view of the sun. We are happy to go with the appearance of things, even though the actuality is somewhat different. Our vantage point has naturally evolved through the body's senses, so the fall into Gaia-centrism and self-centeredness is easily understood and forgivable. It is what we might call the conventional subject-object view of the world. It is not entirely true, but overall, it works pretty well, as far as it goes. This same impulse to make a center and place ourselves in it colors virtually everything we see and do, and so it is no wonder that it also affects even our experience of awareness, at least until we peel back the conventional view we impose on ourselves, and experience it as it actually is.

Our point of view stems inevitably from our point of viewing.

Since our experience is centered on the body, everything that is apprehended seems to be in relationship to its location, and known through the senses. There is the seer and what is seen, the smeller and what is smelled, the taster and what is tasted, in a word, the observer and the observed. There seems to be a natural separation between the two, which is so self-evident that it is hardly ever questioned or explored except by philosophers. When we begin the practice of mindfulness, that invariable sense of separation, expressed as the separation between the observer and what is being observed, continues. We feel as if we are watching our breath as if it is separate from whoever is doing the observing. We watch our thoughts. We watch our feelings, as if there were a real entity in here, a "me" who is carrying out the instructions, doing the watching, and experiencing the results. We never dream that there may be observation without an observer, that is until we naturally, without any forcing, fall into observing, attending, apprehending, knowing. In other words, until we fall into awareness. When we do, even for the briefest of moments, there can be an experience of all separation between subject and object evaporating. There is knowing without a knower, seeing without a seer, thinking without a thinker, more like impersonal phenomena merely unfolding in awareness. The viewing platform centered on the self, and therefore self-centered in the most basic of ways, dissolves when we actually rest in awareness, in the knowing itself. This is simply a property of awareness, and of mind, just as it is for space. It doesn't mean that we are no longer a person, just that the boundaries and the repertoire of being a person have dramatically expanded, and are no longer limited to the separation we conventionally inhabit that has me in here and the world out there, and everything centered on me as agent, as observer, even as meditator.

The larger, less self-oriented view emerges as we venture beyond the conventional boundaries of our five senses into the landscape, or should I say "spacescape" or "mindscape" of awareness itself, or what we might call "pure" awareness. It is something we have all already tasted to one degree or another in some moments, however brief, even if we have never been involved with meditating in any formal sense. But the degree to which we can inhabit a subjectless, objectless, non-dual awareness (where there would no longer be an "us" who is "inhabiting" anything) increases as we give ourselves over wholeheartedly to attending. It can also be revealed to us suddenly in moments when conditions are ripe for it, often catalyzed by intense pain, or, more rarely, by intense joy. The I-centeredness falls away, there is no longer a center or a periphery to awareness. There is simply knowing, seeing, feeling, sensing, thinking, feeling.

We have all tasted the boundarylessness of awareness on those occasions when we were able to suspend our own point of view momentarily and see from another person's point of view and feel with him or her. We call this feeling empathy. If we are too self-absorbed and caught up in our own experience in any moment, we will be unable to shift our perspective in this way and won't even think to try. When we are self-preoccupied, there is virtually no awareness of whole domains of reality we may be living immersed in every day but which nevertheless are continually impinging on and influencing our lives. Our emotions, and particularly the intensely afflictive emotions that "sweep us away," such as anger, fear, and sadness, can all too easily blind us to the full picture of what is actually happening with others and within ourselves.

Such unawareness has its own inevitable consequences. Why are we sometimes so surprised when things fall apart in a relationship when our own self-centeredness may have been starving it of oxygen for years while preventing us from seeing and knowing what was right beneath our noses the whole time?

Since awareness at first blush seems to be a subjective experience, it is hard for us not to think that we are the subject, the thinker, the feeler, the seer, the doer and as such, the very center of the universe, the very center of the field of our awareness. Perceiving thus, we take everything in the universe, or at least our universe, quite personally.

Awareness can feel as if it expands out in all directions from a center localized within us. Therefore, it feels as if it is "my" awareness. But that is a trick our senses play on us, just as with the feeling that everything in the universe is in relationship to our location because we happen to be here looking out. In one way, perhaps awareness *is* centered on us, in that we are a localized node of receptivity. In more fundamental ways, it is not. Awareness is without center or periphery, like space itself.

Awareness is also non-conceptual before thinking splits experience into subject and object. It is empty and so can contain everything, including thought. It is boundless. And above all, amazingly, it is knowing.

The Tibetans call this fundamental quality of knowing "mind essence." Cognitive neuroscientists call it sentience. As we have seen, no one understands it. In some ways, we know it is dependent on neurons, on brain architecture, and the infinite number of possible neuronal connections because you can lose it with certain kinds of brain damage, and because animals seem to have it as well to varying degrees. In other ways, we may just be describing the necessary properties of a receiver that allows us to tap into a field of potentiality that was here from the beginning... for the very fact of our consciousness means the potential for such was here from the beginning, whatever "beginning" might mean.

In other words, knowing has always been possible because otherwise, we wouldn't be here to know. This is the so-called anthropic principle, invoked by cosmologists in their dialogues about origins and possible multiple universes. Speaking modestly, we might say that we are at least one avenue this universe has developed for knowing itself, to whatever degree that might be possible, even though there is no volition involved or cosmic "need" for evolution or consciousness.

With such an inheritance, it might be useful to explore the apparent boundaries of our knowing of ourselves, not as separate from nature, but as a seamlessly embedded expression of it. What greater adventure is there than to adventure in the field of awareness, of sentience itself? Just because science suggests that our awareness— as Steven Pinker puts it in his book *How the Mind Works,* "the most undeniable thing there is" [although it is not a thing]—might be forever beyond our conceptual grasp, that should not deter us in the slightest.

For there are ways of knowing that go beyond conceptualizing and some that come before conceptualizing. When awareness experiences itself, new dimensions of possibility open up.

We can dramatically increase the likelihood of awareness experiencing itself through the intentional cultivation of mindfulness, by learning to pay attention non-conceptually and non-judgmentally, as if it really mattered—because it does.

EMPTINESS

I'm Nobody! Who are you?
Are you—Nobody—Too?
Then there's a pair of us?
Don't tell! they'd advertise—you know!

How dreary—to be—Somebody!
How public—like a Frog—
To tell one's name—the livelong June—
To an admiring Bog!

EMILY DICKINSON

A rabbi during high-holiday services was overcome with a sense of oneness and connectedness with the universe and with God. Transported in a sudden state of ecstasy, he exclaimed, "O Lord, I am your servant. You are everything, I am nothing." The cantor, deeply moved in his heart, exclaimed in turn, "O Lord, I am nothing." Then the janitor of the synagogue, deeply moved himself, was heard to exclaim, "O Lord, I am nothing," at which the rabbi leaned over to the cantor and whispered, "Look who thinks he's nothing."

And so it goes in our perpetual attempts to define ourselves as somebodies rather than nobodies, perhaps suspecting deep down that we really are nobodies and that our lives, no matter what our accomplishments, are built on shifting sands, with no firm foundation, or perhaps no ground at all. Robert Fuller, in a highly elegant analysis in the book *Somebodies and Nobodies*, sees this tension in ourselves and between each other as the fundamental motive force behind the social and political ills of violence, racism, sexism, fascism, anti-Semitism, and ageism plaguing the world. His solution? What he calls "dignitarianism," that we treat everyone as having the same fundamental dignity that transcends their standing and accomplishments, which are, he argues cogently, as does Jared Diamond in *Guns, Germs, and Steel*, in large part more a matter of accident, opportunity, and geography than anything else. Harvard AIDS public health researcher Jonathan Mann, who died in the Swissair Flight 111 crash off the coast of Nova Scotia, himself a tireless advocate for the role of dignity in creating and sustaining health on all levels in our world, wrote: "Injuries to individual and collective dignity may represent a hitherto unrecognized pathogenic force with a destructive capacity toward physical, mental, and social well-being equal to that of viruses or bacteria." Powerful words.

We human beings are indeed all geniuses of one kind or another, and what we hunger for most, and what most requires protecting it seems, is our fundamental dignity. "It turns out," writes Fuller, "that what people need and want is not to dominate others, but to be recognized by them." It's an interesting thought. Diamond would no doubt disagree, given the endlessly repeated history of domination of more technologically advanced cultures over less technically advanced ones.

Yet for all our desire for recognition, to be seen and known and accepted as we are, and to have that be recognized as a basic human right, how easily we can be caught by our own limited and self-centered thinking, even when it is so-called "spiritual" thinking, perhaps, especially when it is so-called spiritual thinking. In the process, we can actually belie and betray what it is we most know, what we most are, and we most care about. Because thinking, when all is said and done, no matter what kind of thinking it is, is still only thinking.

Who do we actually think we are? "Look who thinks he's nothing!" And *what* do we think we are? These are questions we shun. We avoid bringing our full intelligence to inquiring into such matters, even though they matter most. We would rather construct a story that emphasizes some aspect of self as a permanent enduring entity, even if you call it "nobody" or "nothing," and then cling to it and feel bad about it, even though we know that we are not really that, than to look into the mysterious nature of our being beyond our names, our appearance, our roles, our accomplishments, our privileges, acknowledged and unacknowledged by us, and our inveterate mind constructions. The habit of making up stories about ourselves that, upon examination, are seen to be only partially true, only true to a degree, makes it very difficult to come to peace of mind, because there is always the lingering sense that we are not entirely who we think we are.

Maybe the fear is that we are less than we think we are, when the actuality of it is that we are much much more.

If we think we are somebody, no matter who we are, we are mistaken. And if we think we are nobody, we are equally mistaken. As Soen Sa Nim might have put it, "If you say you are somebody, you are attached to name and form, so I will hit you thirty times. If you say you are nobody, you are attached to emptiness, so I will hit you thirty times. What can you do?"

Perhaps it is thinking itself that is the problem here.

Joko Beck, a cherished American Zen teacher and friend who died at age 94 in 2011, opened her book *Nothing Special* with a powerful image emphasizing the transitory and fleeting character of our lives as individual entities in the larger stream of life:

We are rather like whirlpools in the river of life. In flowing forward, a river or stream may hit many rocks, branches, or irregularities in the ground, causing whirlpools to spring up spontaneously here and there. Water entering one whirlpool quickly passes through and rejoins the river, eventually joining another whirlpool and moving on. Though for short periods, it seems to be distinguishable as a separate event, the water in the whirlpools is just the river itself. The stability of a whirlpool is only temporary... However, we want to think that this little whirlpool that we are isn't part of the stream. We want to see ourselves as permanent and stable. Our whole energy goes into trying to protect our supposed separateness. To protect the separateness, we set up artificial, fixed boundaries; as a consequence, we accumulate excess baggage, stuff that slips into our whirlpool and can't flow out again. So things clog up our whirlpool and the process gets messy... Neighboring whirlpools may get less water because of our frantic holding on...

There is significant benefit and freedom in allowing ourselves to recognize how impersonal the process of life really is, and how readily, out of fear and out of thinking, we reify it into the personal in an absolutist sort of way and then get stuck inside constraining boundaries that are of our own creation, nothing more. We are a culture of nouns. We turn things into things, and we do the same with non-things, like whirlpools and awareness, and who we are. This is where we unwittingly become attached to name and form. We need to watch out above all for our relationship to the personal pronouns. Otherwise, we will automatically take things personally when they really aren't at all, and in the process miss, or mis-take, what actually is.

As we noted back in the chapter "No Attachments," the Buddha once famously said that all of his teachings could be condensed into one sentence, "Nothing is to be clung to as 'I,' 'me,' or 'mine.'" It brings up the immediate question of identity and self-identification, and our habit of reifying, that is concretizing, the personal pronoun into an absolute and unexamined "self" and then living inside that "story of me" for a lifetime without examining its accuracy or completeness. In Buddhism, this reification is seen as the root of all suffering, delusion, and afflictive emotions, a mis-identifying of the totality of one's being with the limited story line we heap on the personal pronoun. This identification occurs without us realizing it or questioning its accuracy. But we can learn to see it and see behind it to a deeper truth, a greater wisdom that is available to us at all times.

*

This emptiness of a solid, enduring locus we can identify and identify with as a self applies to a whole host of processes, from politics to business to our own biology. Take a business example. "It's the process," businesspeople often say, "not the product, which is most important." "Care for the process and the product will take care of itself," meaning, I suppose, that a good product will emerge out of a process that keeps the essentials in mind on multiple levels, including the purpose of the process.

Another way people put it is that, in business, you need to keep in mind what business you are in. The standard business school example: Are you in the airlines business, or the business of moving people safely and happily to where they want to go? The former might tend to focus on the limitations of the planes, scheduling, safety, and so on, and wind up with a lot of excuses for why they can't do any better, and why the quality of the service, including cancellations and delays and the food, and the flow of information back to customers is often so dismal. The latter might subtly or not so subtly change how one saw the obstacles to customer satisfaction, and mobilize creative new ways of imagining and galvanizing the wherewithal (i.e., the planes, the ticket counters, the baggage handling, the scheduling, all the employees) to accomplish the mission via a more effective, competitive, and profitable process. In any event, it is a nod to the fact that process is intimately related to product or outcome or dynamic. Ultimately, as they say, it is the people who make the business. Yet, whether it is the for-profit world or the non-profit organization, you still need the business plan, and it has to be good. What that is is a story unto itself for any and every business.

All the same, what "the business" is is hard to put one's finger on. In a way, it is not the employers, not the employees, not the suppliers, not the customers, not the products. It is the entire continually morphing interactive, interconnected process. You won't find "the business" in any of its parts. It is empty, you might say, of any inherent existence. And yet, when it works, it works. On the conventional level, this process that is at its core empty of self-existence, can make things happen, improve people's lives, be traded on the floor of the stock exchange. But it may be a healthier process if all aspects of the business, including its intrinsic emptiness, are held in awareness and taken into account as appropriate.

To take a biological example, life itself is a process too, and a lot more complex than an airline, or any other business. Take your own body. The thirty trillion or so "employees," your body's cells (to say nothing of the estimated sixty trillion or so bacteria that make up the microbiome colonizing your body) are continually in process, each hopefully and amazingly doing what it is supposed to be doing, so that bone cells don't think they are liver cells, and heart cells don't think they are nerve cells or kidney cells, even though they all have the potential, the blueprints and instructional sets stashed away somewhere in the "stacks" of their chromosome libraries, to do all those other "jobs." But the funny thing is, though, if you stop and think about it for a minute, strictly speaking none of those trillions of citizens of your body are working for "you." It is all rather impersonal. Your cells are just doing what they do, following their nature as laid down in the genetic code and in the historical continuity of cell-based life going all the way back.

What we think of as our unique personhood is mysteriously the product of that process, just as any business enterprise is a product of its own energies and processes and output. Our body and its health, our sentience, our emotions are all intimately dependent on our biochemistry: on ion channels, axonal transport, protein synthesis and degradation, enzymatic catalysis and metabolism, DNA replication and repair, regulation of cell division and gene expression, immunosurveillance through macrophages and lymphocytes, genetically programmed and highly regulated cell death (technically known as apoptosis), antibody production to neutralize and dispel compounds and structures the body has never seen before that might be harmful. The list of complex cellular processes and their seamless integration into a society we call the living organism is a long one, and even now, for all our knowledge, still far from complete.

And that process, when you look deeply into it, is also somehow empty of any fixed, enduring selfhood. There is no "us," no "somebody" in it that can be identified, no matter how hard we look. We are not in our ribosomes or our mitochondria, not in our bones or our skin, not in our brains, though our experience of being a person and living a life and interfacing with a world are all dependent on at least a minimal level of functioning and coherence of all of that on levels we are still hard pressed to imagine, for all our scientific precocity and brilliance.

Nor are we our eyes. A great deal is known about vision, yet we do not know how we create the world we live in from the light coming into our eyes. We have an experience of the sky being blue on a clear day, yet there is no "blueness" to be found either in the light of that particular wavelength nor in the retina, the optic nerves, or in the occipital cortex that is the visual center of the brain. And yet we experience the sky instantly as blue. Where does the experiencing of "blue" come from? How does it arise?

We don't know. It is a mystery, as is every other phenomenon that emerges through our senses, including our mind and our sense of being a separately existing self. Our senses build a world for us and situate us within it. This constructed world usually has a high degree of coherence, and a strong sense of there being a perceiver and whatever is being perceived, a thinker and whatever is being thought, a feeler and whatever is being felt. It is all impersonal process, and if there can be said to be a product, it is nowhere to be found in the parts themselves.

Of course, we are one of evolution's solutions to getting around on the planet in successful ways as a species. Just like spiders, and earthworms, and toads. We are well adapted to the challenges of living by our wits rather than merely by our instincts, although that is not to denigrate our instincts in the slightest. We have opposable thumbs at our disposal, and an upright bipedal gait that frees our hands to grasp things and to fabricate tools and gadgets. Importantly, we also have thought and awareness at our disposal, at least as inherent capabilities that can be refined and used for multiple purposes under rapidly changing conditions.

Scientists call these characteristics *emergent phenomena*. Ursula Goodenough, a masterful biologist and teacher at Washington University in St. Louis, cleverly speaks of them as "something more from nothing but." Emergent properties do just that. They emerge as forms and patterns that come out of the complexity of the process itself. They are not attributable to the individual parts of the process, but to the interactions among the parts. And they are not predictable in any detail either. They lie on what is called "the edge of chaos." No complexity, no chaos, and you have a very ordered and predictable system, like a stone or a long-dead body. Too high a degree of chaos in a dynamical system, and you get disorder, dis-regulation, dis-ease, and symptoms of that dis-regulation such as atrial fibrillation or panic attacks. There is a lack of overriding coherence or order. In between, you get the interesting stuff.

A living, dynamical system at the edge of chaos is always, well... at the edge of chaos, conjuring what seems in one way to be quite a delicate balance, in another way, a process that seems remarkably robust, with a complex and continually changing order of its own that keeps it fairly stable. Think of a rhinoceros, a life form threatened with impending extinction. What an extraordinary manifestation, so well adapted to its environment, when it had one that was unthreatened by forces beyond its ken. Its very existence, the dynamical balance and complexity of impersonal life processes, the mystery of the whole of it, its very form and function giving rise to something beyond form and function, to an emergence of sentience, to rhinoceros mind, living within its own coherence on its own terms, completely embedded in and wholly integrated into its own natural rhinoceros world, yet empty of any inherent existence as an isolated self, a "whirlpool" in the stream of life. This is what makes life so interesting. And, we might add, sacred. And important to protect and honor.

Emergent phenomena are not restricted to living systems. Chess is in essence not the pieces or the moves, but what emerges when highly skilled players interact with the rules of the game. Knowing the rules doesn't give you chess. Chess is tasted in the playing, when you really know that universe through total immersion and the interplay of minds, a set of agreed-upon rules, and the board and pieces, and the possibility of learning. None by itself is chess. All are needed for chess to emerge. Same for baseball, or any other sport. We love to see what emerges, again and again, and again, because you never know. That's why the game has to be *played*.

The Heart Sutra, chanted by Mahayana Buddhists around the world, intones:

Form does not differ from emptiness, emptiness does not differ from form. That which is form is emptiness, that which is emptiness, form. The same is true for feelings, perceptions, impulses, consciousness.

People can get scared even hearing such a thing, and may think that it is nihilistic. But it is not nihilistic at all. Emptiness means empty of inherent self-existence, in other words, that nothing, no person, no business, no nation, no atom, exists in and of itself as an enduring entity, isolated, absolute, independent of everything else. Nothing! Everything emerges out of the complex play of particular causes and conditions that are themselves always changing.

This is a tremendous insight into the nature of reality. And it was arrived at long before quantum physics and complexity theory, through direct non-conceptual meditative practices, not through thinking or mere philosophizing.

Think of it. That new car you are so excited about. A whirlpool, nothing more. Empty. Soon to be on the junk pile. In the interim, to be enjoyed, but not clung to. Same for our bodies. Same for other people. We make so much of people, we reify them as deities or devils, tell ourselves big stories or little stories of their triumphs or tragedies, divide them into somebodies and nobodies, but they and all of us are soon gone, for all the trouble we caused or the beauty we brought into the world. The big issues of yesterday are literally nothing today. The big issues of today will be nothing tomorrow. That doesn't mean they were not or are not important. In fact, they may be far more important than we can possibly conceive. Therefore, we need to be ultracareful not to turn them into a kind of mindless fodder for consumption by thought alone. If we realize the emptiness of things, then we will simultaneously realize their gravity, their fullness, their interconnectedness, and that may cause us to act with greater purpose and greater integrity, and perhaps as well with greater wisdom in our private lives and also in the shaping of our national policies and conduct as a body politic on the world stage.

In fact, it is helpful to recognize the intrinsic emptiness of what may seem like an enduring self-existence in any and all phenomena, and at all times. It could free us, individually and collectively, of our clinging to small-minded self-serving interests and desires, and ultimately to all clinging. It could also free us from small-minded self-serving actions so often driven by unwise perceptions or outright mis-perception of what is occurring in either inner or outer land-scapes. That is not to suggest any kind of immoral passivity or quiescence, but rather a wise and compassionate awareness that keeps the inherent non-existing emptiness of self in mind, and is not afraid to act forcefully and wholeheartedly out of that understanding and see what happens.

For emptiness is intimately related to fullness. Emptiness doesn't mean a meaningless void, an occasion for nihilism, passivity, and despair or an abandoning of human values. On the contrary, emptiness is fullness, means fullness, allows for fullness, is the invisible, intangible "space" within which discrete events can emerge and unfold. No emptiness, no fullness. It's as simple as that. Emptiness points to the interconnectedness of all things, processes and phenomena. Emptiness allows for a true ethics, based on reverence for life and the recognition of the interconnectedness of all things and the folly of forcing things to fit one's own small-minded and shortsighted models for maximizing one's own advantage when there is no fixed enduring you to benefit from it, whether "you" is referring to an individual or a country.

The sutra drones on:

> No eyes, no ears, no nose, no tongue, no body, no mind, no color, no sound, no smell, no taste, no touch, no object of mind, no realm of eyes and so forth until no realm of mind consciousness.

Look what it is doing with the senses, with our gateways for knowing the world!

It is reminding us that none of our senses or what is sensed has any absolute independent existence. They are all part of a larger fabric of causes and events woven together. We need this re-minding over and over again to break or at least call into question the persistent habit of believing that the appearance of things is the reality.

No ignorance and also no extinction of it and so forth until
no old age and death and also no extinction of them.

Here the sutra is reminding us that all our concepts are empty
of intrinsic self-existence, including our views of ourselves and our
possibilities for improving and transcending anything. It is pointing to the non-dual, beyond all thinking, beyond all limiting concepts, including all Buddhist teachings, which here, and in the
coming lines, are being explicitly included as having no intrinsic self-
existence:

No suffering, no origination, no stopping, no path, no cognition, also no attainment with nothing to attain.

The Four Noble Truths, the Eightfold Path...all out the window. And yet, and yet...

The Bodhisattva depends on Prajna Paramita and the mind is
no hindrance; without any hindrance no fears exist. Far apart
from every perverted view she dwells in Nirvana.
      In the three worlds all Buddhas depend on Prajna Param-
ita and attain Anuttara Samyak Sambodhi.

Once we recognize, remember, and embody in the way we hold
the moment and the way we live our lives that there is no attainment and
nothing to attain, the sutra is saying all attainment is possible. This is
the gift of emptiness, the practice of the non-dual, the manifestation
of prajna paramita, of supreme perfect wisdom. And we already have
it. All that is required is to be it. When we recognize that we already
are, then form is form, and emptiness is emptiness. And the mind
is no longer caught, in anything. It is no longer self-centered. It is
free.

*

I said to the wanting-creature inside me:
What is this river you want to cross?
There are no travelers on the river-road, and no road.
Do you see anyone moving about on the bank, or resting?
There is no river at all, and no boat, and no boatman.
There is no towrope either, and no one to pull it.
There is no ground, no sky, no time, no bank, no ford!

And there is no body, and no mind!
Do you believe there is some place that will make the soul less thirsty?
In that great absence you will find nothing.

Be strong then, and enter into your own body;
there you have a solid place for your feet,
Think about it carefully!
Don't go off somewhere else!

Kabir says this: just throw away all thoughts of imaginary things,
and stand firm in that which you are.

KABIR
Translated by Robert Bly

"There is no spoon." Line from the movie, *The Matrix*

You live in illusions and the appearance of things.
There is a Reality, you are that Reality.
When you recognize this you will realize that you are nothing,
and being nothing, you are everything. That is all.

KALU RINPOCHE, TIBETAN LAMA

ACKNOWLEDGMENTS

Since the origins of these four volumes go back a long way, there are a number of people to whom I wish to express my gratitude and indebtedness for their many contributions at various stages of the writing and publishing of these books.

For the initial volume, published in 2005, I would like to thank my dharma brother, Larry Rosenberg of the Cambridge Insight Meditation Center, as well as Larry Horwitz, and my father-in-law, the late Howard Zinn, for reading the entire manuscript back in the day and sharing their keen and creative insights with me. My thanks as well to Alan Wallace, Arthur Zajonc, Doug Tanner, and Richard Davidson and to Will Kabat-Zinn and Myla Kabat-Zinn for reading portions of the manuscript and giving me their wise council and feedback. I also thank the original publisher, Bob Miller, and the original editor, Will Schwalbe, now both at Flatiron Books, for their support and friendship, then and now.

Deep and special appreciation, gratitude, and indebtedness to my editor of the four new volumes, Michelle Howry, executive editor at Hachette Books, and to Lauren Hummel and the entire Hachette team that worked so cooperatively and effectively on this series. Working with you, Michelle, has been an absolute pleasure at every stage of this adventure. I so appreciate the gentle collegiality, your care and attention to high-resolution detail in every regard, and you skillfully keeping all the moving pieces of this project on track.

While I have received support, encouragement, and advice from many, of course any inaccuracies or shortcomings in the text are entirely my own.

I wish to express enduring gratitude and respect to all my teaching colleagues, past and present in the Stress Reduction Clinic and the Center for Mindfulness and, more recently, also to those teachers and researchers who are part of the CFM's global network of affiliate institutions. All have literally and metaphorically dedicated their lives and their passion to this work. At the time of the original book, those who had taught MBSR in the Stress Reduction Clinic for varying periods of time from 1979 to 2005 were Saki Santorelli, Melissa Blacker, Florence Meleo-Meyer, Elana Rosenbaum, Ferris Buck Urbanowski, Pamela Erdmann, Fernando de Torrijos, James Carmody, Danielle Levi Alvares, George Mumford, Diana Kamila, Peggy Roggenbuck-Gillespie, Debbie Beck, Zayda Vallejo, Barbara Stone, Trudy Goodman, Meg Chang, Larry Rosenberg, Kasey Carmichael, Franz Moekel, the late Ulli Kesper-Grossman, Maddy Klein, Ann Soulet, Joseph Koppel, the late Karen Ryder, Anna Klegon, Larry Pelz, Adi Bemak, Paul Galvin, and David Spound.

In 2018, my admiration and gratitude go to the current teachers in the Center for Mindfulness and its affiliate programs: Florence Meleo-Meyers, Lynn Koerbel, Elana Rosenbaum, Carolyn West, Bob Stahl, Meg Chang, Zayda Vallejo, Brenda Fingold, Dianne Horgan, Judson Brewer, Margaret Fletcher, Patti Holland, Rebecca Eldridge, Ted Meissner, Anne Twohig, Ana Arrabe, Beth Mulligan, Bonita Jones, Carola Garcia, Gustavo Diex, Beatriz Rodriguez, Melissa Tefft, Janet Solyntjes, Rob Smith, Jacob Piet, Claude Maskens, Charlotte Borch-Jacobsen, Christiane Wolf, Kate Mitcheom, Bob Linscott, Laurence Magro, Jim Colosi, Julie Nason, Lone Overby Fjorback, Dawn MacDonald, Leslie Smith Frank, Ruth Folchman, Colleen Camenisch, Robin Boudette, Eowyn Ahlstrom, Erin Woo, Franco Cuccio, Geneviève Hamelet, Gwenola Herbette, and Ruth Whitall. Florence Meleo-Meyer and Lynn Koerbel have been outstanding leaders and nurturers of the global network of MBSR teachers at the CFM.

Profound appreciation to all those who contributed so critically in so many different ways to the administration of the MBSR Clinic and the Center for Mindfulness in Medicine, Health Care, and Society and to their various research and clinical endeavors from the very beginning: Norma Rosiello, Kathy Brady, Brian Tucker, Anne Skillings, Tim Light, Jean Baril, Leslie Lynch, Carol Lewis, Leigh Emery, Rafaela Morales, Roberta Lewis, Jen Gigliotti, Sylvia Ciario, Betty Flodin, Diane Spinney, Carol Hester, Carol Mento, Olivia Hobletzell, the late Narina Hendry, Marlene Samuelson, Janet Parks, Michael Bratt, Marc Cohen, and Ellen Wingard; and in the current era, building on a robust platform developed under the leadership of Saki Santorelli over seventeen years, I extend my gratitude to the current leadership of Judson Brewer, Dianne Horgan, Florence Meleo-Meyer, and Lynn Koerbel, with amazing support from Jean Baril, Jacqueline Clark, Tony Maciag, Ted Meissner, Jessica Novia, Maureen Titus, Beverly Walton, Ashley Gladden, Lynne Littizzio, Nicole Rocijewicz and Jean Welker. And a deep bow to Judson Brewer, MD, PhD, who became, in 2017, the founding director of the Division of Mindfulness in the Department of Medicine at the University of Massachusetts Medical School—the first division of mindfulness in a medical school in the world, and very much a sign of the times and of the promise of things to come.

On the research side of the CFM in 2018, robust appreciation for the breadth and depth of your work and contributions: Judson Brewer, Remko van Lutterveld, Prasanta Pal, Michael Datko, Andrea Ruf, Susan Druker, Ariel Beccia, Alexandra Roy, Hanif Benoit, Danny Theisen, and Carolyn Neal.

Finally, I would also like to express my gratitude and respect for the thousands of people everywhere around the world who work in or are researching mindfulness-based approaches in medicine, psychiatry, psychology, health care, education, the law, social justice, refugee healing in the face of trauma and sometimes genocide (as in South Darfur), childbirth and parenting, the workplace, government, prisons, and other facets of society, and who take care to honor the dharma in its universal depth and beauty in doing so. You know who you are, whether you are named here or not! And if you are not, it is only due to my own shortcomings and the limits of space. I want to explicitly honor the work of Paula Andrea Ramirez Diazgranados in Columbia and South Darfur; Hui Qi Tong in the U.S. and China; Kevin Fong, Roy Te Chung Chen, Tzungkuen Wen, Helen Ma, Jin Mei Hu, and Shih Shih Ming in China, Taiwan, and Hong Kong; Heyoung Ahn in Korea; Junko Bickel and Teruro Shiina in Japan; Leena Pennenen in Finland; Simon Whitesman and Linda Kantor in South Africa; Claude Maskens, Gwénola Herbette, Edel Max, Caroline Lesire, and Ilios Kotsou in Belgium; Jean-Gérard Bloch, Geneviève Hamelet, Marie-Ange Pratili, and Charlotte Borch-Jacobsen in France; Katherine Bonus, Trish Magyari, Erica Sibinga, David Kearney, Kurt Hoelting, Carolyn McManus, Mike Brumage, Maureen Strafford, Amy Gross, Rhonda Magee, George Mumford, Carl Fulwiler, Maria Kluge, Mick Krasner, Trish Luck, Bernice Todres, Ron Epstein, and Representative Tim Ryan in the U.S.: Paul Grossman, Maria Kluge, Sylvia Wiesman-Fiscalini, Linda Hehrhaupt, and Petra Meibert in Germany; Joke Hellemans, Johan Tinge, and Anna Speckens in Holland; Beatrice Heller and Regula Saner in Switzerland; Rebecca Crane, Willem Kuyken, John Teasdale, Mark Williams, Chris Cullen, Richard Burnett, Jamie Bristow, Trish Bartley, Stewart Mercer, Chris Ruane, Richard Layard, Guiaume Hung, and Ahn Nguyen in the UK; Zindel Segal and Norm Farb in Canada; Gabor Fasekas in Hungary; Macchi dela Vega in Argentina; Johan Bergstad, Anita Olsson, Angeli Holmstedt; Ola Schenström, Camilla Sköld in Sweden; Andries Kroese in Norway; Jakob Piet and Lone Overby Fjorback in Denmark; and Franco Cuccio in Italy. May your work continue to reach those who are most in need of it, touching, clarifying, and nurturing what is deepest and best in us all, and thus contributing, in ways little and big to the healing and transformation that humanity so sorely longs for and aspires to.

Mindfulness Meditation

Analayo, B. *Satipatthana: The Direct Path to Realization*, Windhorse, Cambridge, UK, 2008.

Beck, C. *Nothing Special: Living Zen*, HarperCollins, San Francisco, 1993.

Buswell, R. B., Jr. *Tracing Back the Radiance: Chinul's Korean Way of Zen*, Kuroda Institute, U of Hawaii Press, Honolulu, 1991.

Goldstein, J. *Mindfulness: A Practical Guide to Awakening*, Sounds True, Boulder, 2013.

Goldstein, J. *One Dharma: The Emerging Western Buddhism*, HarperCollins, San Francisco, 2002.

Hanh, T. N. *The Heart of the Buddha's Teachings*, Broadway, New York, 1998.

Hanh, T. N. *How to Love*, Parallax Press, Berkeley, 2015

Hanh, T. N. *How to Sit*, Parallax Press, Berkeley, 2014.

Hanh, T. N. *The Miracle of Mindfulness*, Beacon, Boston, 1976.

Kapleau, P. *The Three Pillars of Zen: Teaching, Practice, and Enlightenment*, Random House, New York, 1965, 2000.

Krishnamurti, J. *This Light in Oneself: True Meditation*, Shambhala, Boston, 1999.

Ricard, M. *Why Meditate?*, Hay House, New York, 2010.

Rosenberg, L. *Breath by Breath: The Liberating Practice of Insight Meditation*, Shambhala, Boston, 1998.

Rosenberg, L. *Living in the Light of Death: On the Art of Being Truly Alive*, Shambhala, Boston, 2000.

Rosenberg, L. *Three Steps to Awakening: A Practice for Bringing Mindfulness to Life*, Shambhala, Boston, 2013.

Salzberg, S. *Lovingkindness*, Shambhala, Boston, 1995.

Salzberg, S. *Real Love: The Art of Mindful Connection*, Flatiron Books, New York, 2017.

Sheng-Yen, C. *Hoofprints of the Ox: Principles of the Chan Buddhist Path*, Oxford University Press, New York, 2001.

Suzuki, S. *Zen Mind, Beginner's Mind*, Weatherhill, New York, 1970.

Thera, N. *The Heart of Buddhist Meditation: The Buddha's Way of Mindfulness*, Red Wheel/Weiser, San Francisco, 1962, 2014.

Treleaven, D. *Trauma-Sensitive Mindfulness: Practices for Safe and Transformative Healing*, W.W. Norton, New York, 2018.

Tulku Urgyen. *Rainbow Painting*, Rangjung Yeshe: Boudhanath, Nepal, 1995.

MBSR

Brandsma, R. *The Mindfulness Teaching Guide: Essential Skills and Competencies for Teaching Mindfulness-Based Interventions*, New Harbinger, Oakland, CA, 2017.

Kabat-Zinn, J. *Full Catastrophe Living: Using the Wisdom of Your Body and Mind to Face Stress, Pain, and Illness*, revised and updated edition, Random House, New York, 2013.

Lehrhaupt, L. and Meibert, P. *Mindfulness-Based Stress Reduction: The MBSR Program for Enhancing Health and Vitality*, New World Library, Novato, CA, 2017.

Rosenbaum, E. *The Heart of Mindfulness-Based Stress Reduction: An MBSR Guide for Clinicians and Clients*, Pesi Publishing, Eau Claire, WI, 2017.

Santorelli, S. *Heal Thy Self: Lessons on Mindfulness in Medicine*, Bell Tower, New York, 1999.

Stahl, B. and Goldstein, E. *A Mindfulness-Based Stress Reduction Workbook*, New Harbinger, Oakland, CA, 2010.

Stahl, B., Meleo-Meyer, F., and Koerbel, L. *A Mindfulness-Based Stress Reduction Workbook for Anxiety*, New Harbinger, Oakland, CA, 2014.

Other Applications of Mindfulness

Bardacke, N. *Mindful Birthing: Training the Mind, Body, and Heart for Childbirth and Beyond*, HarperCollins, New York, 2012.

Bartley, T. *Mindfulness: A Kindly Approach to Cancer*, Wiley-Blackwell, West Sussex, UK, 2016.

Bartley, T. *Mindfulness-Based Cognitive Therapy for Cancer*, Wiley-Blackwell, West Sussex, UK, 2012.

Bays, J. C. *Mindful Eating: A Guide to Rediscovering a Healthy and Joyful Relationship with Food*, Shambhala, Boston, 2009, 2017.

Bays, J. C. *Mindfulness on the Go: Simple Meditation Practices You Can Do Anywhere*, Shambhala, Boston, 2014.

Biegel, G. *The Stress-Reduction Workbook for Teens: Mindfulness Skills to Help You Deal with Stress*, New Harbinger, Oakland, CA, 2017.

Brewer, Judson. *The Craving Mind: From Cigarettes to Smartphones to Love—Why We Get Hooked and How We Can Break Bad Habits*, Yale, New Haven, 2017

Brown, K. W., Creswell, J. D., and Ryan, R. M. (eds). *Handbook of Mindfulness: Theory, Research, and Practice*, Guilford, New York, 2015.

Carlson, L. and Speca, M. *Mindfulness-Based Cancer Recovery: A Step-by-Step MBSR Approach to Help You Cope with Treatment and Reclaim Your Life*, New Harbinger, Oakland, CA, 2010.

Cullen, M. and Pons, G. B. *The Mindfulness-Based Emotional Balance Workbook: An Eight-Week Program for Improved Emotion Regulation and Resilience*, New Harbinger, Oakland, CA, 2015.

Epstein, R. *Attending: Medicine, Mindfulness, and Humanity*, Scribner, New York, 2017.

Germer, C. *The Mindful Path to Self-Compassion*, Guilford, New York, 2009.

Goleman, G, and Davidson, R. J. *Altered Traits: Science Reveals How Meditation Changes Your Mind, Brain, and Body*, Avery/Random House, New York, 2017.

Gunaratana, B. H. *Mindfulness in Plain English*, Wisdom, Somerville, MA, 2002.

Jennings, P. *Mindfulness for Teachers: Simple Skills for Peace and Productivity in the Classroom*, W.W. Norton, New York, 2015.

Kaiser-Greenland, S. *The Mindful Child*, Free Press, New York, 2010.

McCown, D., Reibel, D., and Micozzi, M. S. (eds.). *Resources for Teaching Mindfulness: An International Handbook*, Springer, New York, 2016.

McCown, D., Reibel, D., and Micozzi, M. S. (eds.). *Teaching Mindfulness: A Practical Guide for Clinicians and Educators*, Springer, New York, 2010.

Penman, D. *The Art of Breathing*, Conari, Newburyport, MA, 2018.

Rechtschaffen, D. *The Mindful Education Workbook: Lessons for Teaching Mindfulness to Students*, W.W. Norton, New York, 2016.

Rechtschaffen, D. *The Way of Mindful Education: Cultivating Wellbeing in Teachers and Students*, W.W. Norton, New York, 2014.

Rosenbaum, E. *Being Well (Even When You Are Sick): Mindfulness Practices for People with Cancer and Other Serious Illnesses*, Shambala, Boston, 2012.

Rosenbaum, E. *Here for Now: Living Well with Cancer Through Mindfulness*, Satya House, Hardwick, MA, 2005.

Segal, Z. V., Williams, J. M. G., and Teasdale, J. D. *Mindfulness-Based Cognitive Therapy for Depression: A New Approach to Preventing Relapse*, second edition, Guilford, New York, 2013.

Teasdale, J. D., Williams, M., and Segal, Z. V. *The Mindful Way Workbook: An Eight-Week Program to Free Yourself from Depression and Emotional Distress*, Guilford, New York, 2014.

Williams, A. K., Owens, R., and Syedullah, J. *Radical Dharma: Talking Race, Love, and Liberation*, North Atlantic Books, Berkeley, 2016.

Williams, J. M. G., Teasdale, J. D., Segal, Z. V., and Kabat-Zinn, J. *The Mindful Way Through Depression: Freeing Yourself from Chronic Unhappiness*, Guilford, New York, 2007.

Williams, M. and Penman, D. *Mindfulness: An Eight-Week Plan for Finding Peace in a Frantic World*, Rhodale, 2012.

Healing

Doidge, N. *The Brain's Way of Healing: Remarkable Discoveries and Recoveries from the Frontiers of Neuroplasticity*, Penguin Random House, New York, 2016.

Goleman, D. *Healing Emotions: Conversations with the Dalai Lama on Mindfulness, Emotions, and Health*, Shambhala, Boston, 1997.

Moyers, B. *Healing and the Mind*, Doubleday, New York, 1993.

Siegel, D. *The Mindful Brain: Reflection and Attunement in the Cultivation of Wellbeing*, W.W. Norton, New York, 2007.

Van der Kolk, B. *The Body Keeps the Score: Brain, Mind, and Body in the Healing of Trauma*, Penguin Random House, New York, 2014.

Poetry

Eliot, T. S. *Four Quartets*, Harcourt Brace, New York, 1943, 1977.

Lao-Tzu, *Tao Te Ching*, (Stephen Mitchell, transl.), HarperCollins, New York, 1988.

Mitchell, S. *The Enlightened Heart*, Harper & Row, New York, 1989.

Oliver, M. *New and Selected Poems*, Beacon, Boston, 1992.

Tanahashi, K. and Leavitt, P. *The Complete Cold Mountain: Poems of the Legendary Hermit, Hanshan*, Shambhala, Boulder, CO, 2018.

Whyte, D. *The Heart Aroused: Poetry and the Preservation of the Soul in Corporate America*, Doubleday, New York, 1994.

Other Books of Interest, Some Mentioned in the Text

Abram, D. *The Spell of the Sensuous*, Vintage, New York, 1996.

Blackburn, E. and Epel, E. *The Telomere Effect: A Revolutionary Approach to Living Younger, Healthier, Longer*, Grand Central Publishing, New York, 2017.

Davidson, R. J., and Begley, S. *The Emotional Life of Your Brain*, Hudson St. Press, New York, 2012.

Harris, Y. N. *Sapiens: A Brief History of Humankind*, HarperCollins, New York, 2015.

Katie, B. and Mitchell, S. *A Mind at Home with Itself*, HarperCollins, New York, 2017.

Luke, H. *Old Age: Journey into Simplicity*, Parabola, New York, 1987.

Montague, A. *Touching: The Human Significance of the Skin*, Harper & Row, New York, 1978.

Pinker, S. *The Better Angels of Our Nature: Why Violence Has Declined*, Penguin Random House, New York, 2012.

Pinker, S. *Enlightenment Now: The Case for Reason, Science, Humanism, and Progress*, Penguin Random House, New York, 2018.

Pinker, S. *How the Mind Works*, W.W. Norton, New York, 1997.

Ricard, M. *Altruism: The Power of Compassion to Change Yourself and the World*, Little Brown, New York, 2013.

Ryan, T. *A Mindful Nation: How a Simple Practice Can Help Us Reduce Stress, Improve Performance, and Recapture the American Spirit*, Hay House, New York, 2012.

Sachs, J. D. *The Price of Civilization: Reawakening American Virtue and Prosperity*, Random House, New York, 2011.

Sachs, O. *The Man Who Mistook His Wife for a Hat*, Touchstone, New York, 1970.

Sachs, O. *The River of Consciousness*, Knopf, New York, 2017.

Sapolsky, R. *Behave: The Biology of Humans at Our Best and Worst*, Penguin Random House, New York, 2017.

Tegmark, M. *The Mathematical Universe: My Quest for the Ultimate Nature of Reality*, Random House, New York, 2014.

Turkle, S. *Alone Together: Why We Expect More from Technology and Less from Each Other*, Basic Books, New York, 2011.

Turkle, S. *Reclaiming Conversation: The Power of Talk in a Digital Age*, Penguin Random House, New York, 2015.

Varela, F. J., Thompson, E., and Rosch, E. *The Embodied Mind: Cognitive Science and Human Experience*, revised edition, MIT Press, Cambridge, MA, 2016.

Wright, R. *Why Buddhism Is True: The Science and Philosophy of Meditation and Enlightenment*, Simon & Schuster, New York, 2017.

Websites

www.umassmed.edu/cfm	Center for Mindfulness, UMass Medical School
www.mindandlife.org	Mind and Life Institute
www.dharma.org	Vipassana retreat centers and schedules

INDEX

Page references in italics indicate quotes or poetry citations.

ABOUT THE AUTHOR

JON KABAT-ZINN, Ph.D., is the founder of MBSR (mindfulness-based stress reduction) and the Stress Reduction Clinic (1979) and of the Center for Mindfulness in Medicine, Health Care, and Society (1995) at the University of Massachusetts Medical School. He is also professor of Medicine emeritus. He leads workshops and retreats on mindfulness for health professionals, the tech and business communities, and for lay audiences worldwide. He is a strong proponent of social justice and economic justice. He is the author or coauthor of ten books, including the bestselling *Wherever You Go, There You Are* and *Full Catastrophe Living*. With his wife Myla Kabat-Zinn, he published a book on mindful parenting, *Everyday Blessings*. He has been featured in numerous documentaries for television around the world, including the PBS Special *Healing and the Mind* with Bill Moyers, *Oprah*, and CBS's *60 Minutes* with Anderson Cooper. He lives in Massachusetts. His work has contributed to a growing movement of mindfulness into mainstream institutions such as medicine, psychology, health care, neuroscience, schools, higher education, business, social justice, criminal justice, prisons, the law, technology, government, and professional sports. Hospitals and medical centers around the world now offer clinical programs based on training in mindfulness and MBSR.

Continue the journey and get the full set of
Jon Kabat-Zinn's four small-but-mighty guides to
mindfulness and meditation, as well as his
bestselling classic *Wherever You Go, There You Are.*

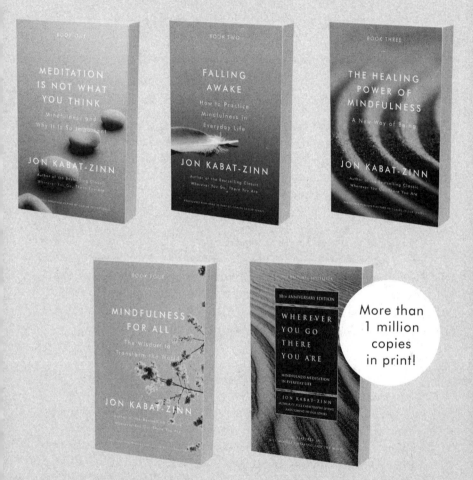

JON KABAT-ZINN, PhD, is the founder of Mindfulness-Based
Stress Reduction (MBSR) and of the Center for Mindfulness in Medicine,
Health Care and Society at the University of Massachusetts, where he
is Professor of Medicine emeritus. He is the author of numerous bestselling books about mindfulness and meditation. For more information,
visit www.jonkabat-zinn.com.

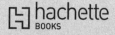

Guided Mindfulness Meditation Practices with Jon Kabat-Zinn

Obtainable as apps, downloads, or CDs
(see below for links)

Series 1

These guided meditations (the body scan and sitting meditation) and guided mindful yoga practices 1 and 2 form the foundational practices of MBSR and are used in MBSR programs around the world. These practices and their use are described in detail in *Full Catastrophe Living*. Each meditation is 45 minutes in length.

Series 2

These guided meditations are designed for people who want a range of shorter guided meditations to help them develop and/or expand and deepen a personal meditation practice based on mindfulness. The series includes the mountain and lake meditations (each 20 minutes) as well as a range of other 10-minute, 20-minute, and 30-minute sitting and lying down practices. This series was originally developed to accompany *Wherever You Go, There You Are*.

Series 3

These guided meditations are designed to accompany this book and the other three volumes based on *Coming to Our Senses*. Series 3 includes guided meditations on the breath and body sensations (breathscape and bodyscape), on sounds (soundscape), thoughts and emotions (mindscape), choiceless awareness (nowscape), and lovingkindness (heartscape), as well as instructions for lying down meditation (corpse pose/dying before you die), mindful walking, and cultivating mindfulness in everyday life (lifescape).

For iPhone and Android apps: www.mindfulnessapps.com

For digital downloads: www.betterlisten.com/pages/jonkabatzinnseries123

For CD sets: www.soundstrue.com/jon-kabat-zinn